NANDA | # NURSING DIAGNOSES:
DEFINITIONS &
CLASSIFICATION

2005–2006

Editorial Committee

Sheila Sparks Ralph, DNSc, RN, FAAN, *Chair*
Martha Craft-Rosenberg, PhD, RN, FAAN
Leann Scroggins, MS, RN
Barbara Vassallo, EdD, RN, CS, ANPC
Judith Warren, PhD, RN, C, FAAN

NANDA

NURSING DIAGNOSES:

DEFINITIONS & CLASSIFICATION

2005–2006

NANDA International
Philadelphia

For information, contact NANDA International, 1211 Locust Street, Philadelphia PA 19107, USA
Telephone: 215.545.7222/800.647.9002
Fax: 215.545.8107
E-mail: NANDA@rmpinc.com
Web site: www.nanda.org

Printed in the United States of America
10 9 8 7 6 5 4 3 2

ISBN 0.9637042-4-9

Contents

Preface

This edition of *NANDA Nursing Diagnoses: Definitions & Classification, 2005–2006,* is published at a time when NANDA International is recognized as a well-established diagnosis terminology. Our terminology has been included in the UMLS and recognized by ANA for quite some time. But more recently it has been HL7 registered, modified to become compatible with ISO, and included in SNOMED-CT. It is also available in several languages, including Chinese, Danish, Dutch, English (U.S. and British), French, German, Icelandic, Italian, Japanese, Norwegian, Portuguese, and Spanish. While there is reason to be proud of our contributions and heritage, change is required for the 21st century.

Changes in this new edition include five new diagnoses, three revised diagnoses, and placement of the NANDA International diagnoses within the NNN Taxonomy of Nursing Practice (see page 252). The new and revised diagnoses reflect increased awareness of the importance of spirituality and religion in health and illness as well as growing global concerns surrounding sedentary lifestyles. The *sedentary lifestyle* diagnosis is significant in another dimension. It was submitted in both English and another language. The Board hopes that many more diagnoses will be submitted in other languages: We are now an international organization, and our diagnoses need to have global relevance for global application.

NANDA International develops terminology to describe the important judgments nurses make in providing nursing care for individuals, families, groups, and communities. These judgments—or diagnoses—are the basis for selection of nursing interventions and outcomes. This relationship speaks to the need for a common structure—or taxonomy. The NNN Taxonomy of Nursing Practice was created and refined over the past 3 years to link nursing diagnoses, interventions, and outcomes (Dochterman & Jones, 2003). It was developed through the NNN Alliance of NANDA International, the Nursing Interventions Classification (NIC), and the Nursing Outcomes Classification (NOC). Contributions from leaders in NANDA International as well as leaders from NIC and NOC are reflected in the Taxonomy of Nursing Practice. The Board welcomes your comments and suggestions, because all classification and taxonomy work is dynamic and constantly changing. Your thoughts are needed to keep it current and useful. Of course, the Taxonomy II of NANDA International is included in this edition. The Taxonomy Committee has made some changes and added diagnoses, but the structure is intact.

Continuing with the pattern in the last edition, all new and revised diagnoses have a "LOE" (level of evidence) number to inform all users of the evidence underlying the diagnoses. The evidence can be found by using the list of three references that best support the diagnoses as a beginning point. Diagnoses must be grounded solidly in evidence. Our policy is clear that critique of diagnoses by members and our Board will include a LOE at the same level or higher than the evidence presented by the diagnosis submitter.

This edition continues to list the diagnoses alphabetically by diagnostic concept to facilitate their ready use. The index also contains an alphabetical listing of diagnoses. For most users this presentation is seen as convenient. We hope you will continue to find it helpful.

This edition is made possible through the hard work of the editorial committee, chaired by Sheila Sparks Ralph. I want to thank each of the editorial committee members and Margo Neal, our editor from Nursecom. Suggestions and feedback from many of you also are included. The Board is committed to continuous refinement and improvement of this book, which is possible with your contributions.

Nursing continues to change rapidly around the world, and our concepts, language, and terms must provide the communication tools needed. I urge all of you to commit to an increase in the scope and comprehensiveness of our diagnoses classification. While the numbers keep slowly increasing, we still have only 172 diagnoses. We need to increase this number.

Nursing language or terminology is the responsibility of nurses. Our responsibility can be met in two ways. First, diagnosis language or terminology work is supported through an organization. If you do not belong, I ask you to join and then to invite ONE other nurse to join our organization. An invitation to join NANDA International is on page 287. The second way to meet our responsibility is to develop or refine ONE diagnosis. Ask yourself what diagnosis you need that is missing. Then, go to www.nlinks.org and examine the concept analysis and diagnosis submission process. Help is available to you from the Diagnosis Review Committee, and I urge you all to get involved. There is nothing more exciting than nursing and describing nursing judgments!

Martha (Marty) Craft-Rosenberg PhD, RN, FAAN
President, NANDA International

Reference

Dochterman, J., & Jones, D. (Eds.). (2003). *Unifying nursing languages: The harmonization of NANDA, NIC, and NOC.* Washington, DC: American Nurses Association.

New nursing diagnoses, 2005

Impaired Religiosity[a]
Readiness for Enhanced Religiosity[a]
Risk for Dysfunctional Grieving[b]
Risk for Impaired Religiosity[a]
Sedentary Lifestyle[c]

Revised diagnoses, 2005

Dysfunctional Grieving[b]
Energy Field Disturbance[d]
Risk for Spiritual Distress[a]

[a] Submitted by Lisa Burkhart, PhD, RN
[b] Submitted by Mary Ann Lavin, ScD, RN, BC, ANP, FAAN
[c] Submitted by Adolf Euirao, RN
[d] Submitted by Rebecca Good, MA, RNC, ACRN, LPC

Introduction

This book is divided into three parts. Part 1 includes the traditional contents of the previous *NANDA Nursing Diagnoses: Definitions & Classification* books — that is, the diagnoses. The diagnoses are listed in *alphabetical order by the diagnostic concept*, not by the first word or descriptor of the diagnosis. Taxonomy II splits the diagnoses into axes (see page 232 for a full explanation). Thus, if you are looking for "impaired wheelchair mobility," you will find it under "mobility," not under "wheelchair" or "impaired."

Part 2 describes the structure of Taxonomy II and how it was developed. Figure 2.1 depicts *Taxonomy II Domains and Classes*; Table 2.1 shows *Taxonomy II: Domains, Classes, and Diagnoses*; and Table 2.2 shows *NNN Taxonomy of Nursing Practice: Placement of Nursing Diagnoses*.

Part 3 includes diagnosis submission guidelines, a process to appeal a decision of the Diagnosis Review Committee on a nursing diagnosis, a glossary, and copyright guidelines; a list of members of the NANDA International Board of Directors, Taxonomy, and Diagnosis Review Committees; NDEC committee members; an invitation to join NANDA; and the index.

How to Use This Book

The nursing diagnoses are listed alphabetically by *diagnostic concept*. For example, *activity intolerance* is listed under "A" because activity is the diagnostic concept. Similarly, *interrupted family process* is listed under "F" because family process is the diagnostic concept.

We hope the organization of *NANDA Nursing Diagnoses: Definitions & Classification 2005–2006* will make it efficient and effective to use. We welcome your feedback. If you have suggestions, please send them to us through the NANDA Web site (http://www.nanda.org) or by calling the office at 800. 647.9002.

Part 1

NANDA NURSING DIAGNOSES 2005–2006

**NANDA Nursing Diagnoses
With Definitions,
Defining Characteristics or
Risk Factors, and Related Factors**

Activity Intolerance
(1982)

Definition *Insufficient physiological or psychological energy to endure or complete required or desired daily activities*

Defining Characteristics
- Verbal report of fatigue or weakness
- Abnormal heart rate or blood pressure response to activity
- Electrocardiographic changes reflecting arrhythmias or ischemia
- Exertional discomfort or dyspnea

Related Factors
Bed rest or immobility
Generalized weakness
Imbalance between oxygen supply/demand
Sedentary lifestyle

RISK FOR ACTIVITY INTOLERANCE
(1982)

Definition *At risk for experiencing insufficient physiological or psychological energy to endure or complete required or desired daily activities*

Risk Factors

Inexperience with the
  activity
Presence of circulatory/
  respiratory problems
History of previous
  intolerance
Deconditioned status

IMPAIRED ADJUSTMENT
(1986, 1998)

Definition *Inability to modify lifestyle/behavior in a manner consistent with a change in health status*

Defining Characteristics

- Denial of health status change
- Failure to take actions that would prevent further health problems
- Failure to achieve optimal sense of control
- Demonstration of nonacceptance of health status change

Related Factors

Low state of optimism
Intense emotional state
Negative attitudes toward health behavior
Absence of intent to change behavior
Multiple stressors
Absence of social support for changed beliefs and practices

Disability or health status change requiring change in lifestyle
Lack of motivation to change behaviors

INEFFECTIVE **A**IRWAY CLEARANCE
(1980, 1996, 1998)

Definition *Inability to clear secretions or obstructions from the respiratory tract to maintain a clear airway*

Defining Characteristics

- Dyspnea
- Diminished breath sounds
- Orthopnea
- Adventitious breath sounds (rales, crackles, rhonchi, wheezes)
- Cough, ineffective or absent
- Sputum production
- Cyanosis
- Difficulty vocalizing
- Wide-eyed
- Changes in respiratory rate and rhythm
- Restlessness

Related Factors

Environmental

  Smoking
  Smoke inhalation
  Second-hand smoke

Obstructed airway

  Airway spasm
  Retained secretions
  Excessive mucus
  Presence of artificial airway
  Foreign body in airway
  Secretions in the bronchi
  Exudate in the alveoli

Physiological

  Neuromuscular dysfunction
  Hyperplasia of the bronchial walls
  Chronic obstructive pulmonary disease
  Infection
  Asthma
  Allergic airways

LATEX ALLERGY RESPONSE
(1998)

Definition   *An allergic response to natural latex rubber products*

Defining Characteristics

Type I Reactions

- Immediate reactions (<1 hour) to latex proteins (can be life threatening)
- Contact urticaria progressing to generalized symptoms
- Edema of the lips, tongue, uvula, and/or throat
- Shortness of breath, tightness in chest, wheezing, bronchospasm leading to respiratory arrest
- Hypotension, syncope, cardiac arrest

May also include:

- Orofacial characteristics
  - Edema of sclera or eyelids
  - Erythema and/or itching of the eyes
  - Tearing of the eyes
  - Nasal congestion, itching, and/or erythema
  - Rhinorrhea
  - Facial erythema

  - Facial itching
  - Oral itching
- Gastrointestinal characteristics
  - Abdominal pain
  - Nausea
- Generalized characteristics
  - Flushing
  - General discomfort
  - Generalized edema
  - Increasing complaint of total body warmth
  - Restlessness

Type IV Reactions

- Delayed onset (hours)
- Eczema
- Irritation
- Reaction to additives (e.g., thiurams, carbamates) causes discomfort
- Redness

Irritant Reactions

- Erythema
- Chapped or cracked skin
- Blisters

Related Factors

No immune mechanism response

RISK FOR LATEX ALLERGY RESPONSE
(1998)

Definition   *At risk for allergic response to natural latex rubber products*

Risk Factors

Multiple surgical procedures, especially from infancy (e.g., spina bifida)

Allergies to bananas, avocados, tropical fruits, kiwi, chestnuts

Professions with daily exposure to latex (e.g., medicine, nursing, dentistry)

Conditions associated with continuous or intermittent catheterization

History of reactions to latex (e.g., balloons, condoms, gloves)

Allergies to poinsettia plants

History of allergies and asthma

Anxiety
(1973, 1982, 1998)

Definition *Vague uneasy feeling of discomfort or dread accompanied by an autonomic response (the source often non-specific or unknown to the individual); a feeling of apprehension caused by anticipation of danger. It is an alerting signal that warns of impending danger and enables the individual to take measures to deal with threat.*

Defining Characteristics

Behavioral
- Diminished productivity
- Scanning and vigilance
- Poor eye contact
- Restlessness
- Glancing about
- Extraneous movement (e.g., foot shuffling, hand/arm movements)
- Expressed concerns due to change in life events
- Insomnia
- Fidgeting

Affective
- Regretful
- Irritability
- Anguish
- Scared
- Jittery
- Overexcited
- Painful and persistent increased helplessness
- Rattled
- Uncertainty
- Increased wariness

- Focus on self
- Feelings of inadequacy
- Fearful
- Distressed
- Worried, apprehensive
- Anxious

Physiological
- Voice quivering
- Trembling/hand tremors
- Shakiness
- Increased respiration (sympathetic)
- Urinary urgency (parasympathetic)
- Increased pulse (sympathetic)
- Pupil dilation (sympathetic)
- Increased reflexes (sympathetic)
- Abdominal pain (parasympathetic)
- Sleep disturbance (parasympathetic)

continued

Anxiety, *continued*

- Tingling in extremities (parasympathetic)
- Cardiovascular excitation (sympathetic)
- Increased perspiration
- Facial tension
- Anorexia (sympathetic)
- Heart pounding (sympathetic)
- Diarrhea (parasympathetic)
- Urinary hesitancy (parasympathetic)
- Fatigue (parasympathetic)
- Dry mouth (sympathetic)
- Weakness (sympathetic)
- Decreased pulse (parasympathetic)
- Facial flushing (sympathetic)
- Superficial vasoconstriction (sympathetic)
- Twitching (sympathetic)
- Decreased blood pressure (parasympathetic)
- Nausea (parasympathetic)
- Urinary frequency (parasympathetic)
- Faintness (parasympathetic)
- Respiratory difficulties (sympathetic)
- Increased blood pressure (sympathetic)

Cognitive

- Blocking of thought
- Confusion
- Preoccupation
- Forgetfulness
- Rumination
- Impaired attention
- Decreased perceptual field
- Fear of unspecified consequences
- Tendency to blame others
- Difficulty concentrating
- Diminished ability to
  - Problem solve
  - Learn
- Awareness of physiologic symptoms

Related Factors

Exposure to toxins
Unconscious conflict
  about essential
  values/goals of life
Familial association/
  heredity
Unmet needs
Interpersonal
  transmission/contagion
Situational/maturational
  crises
Threat of death

Threat to self-concept
Stress
Substance abuse
Threat to or change in
– Role status
– Health status
– Interaction patterns
– Role function
– Environment
– Economic status

DEATH ANXIETY
(1998)

Definition *Apprehension, worry, or fear related to death or dying*

Defining Characteristics

- Worrying about the impact of one's own death on significant others
- Powerless over issues related to dying
- Fear of loss of physical and/or mental abilities when dying
- Anticipated pain related to dying
- Deep sadness
- Fear of the process of dying
- Concerns of overworking the caregiver as terminal illness incapacitates self
- Concern about meeting one's creator or feeling doubtful about the existence of a God or Higher Being
- Total loss of control over any aspect of one's own death
- Negative death images or unpleasant thoughts about any event related to death or dying
- Fear of delayed demise
- Fear of premature death because it prevents the accomplishment of important life goals
- Worrying about being the cause of other's grief and suffering
- Fear of leaving family alone after death
- Fear of developing a terminal illness
- Denial of one's own mortality or impending death

Related Factors

To be developed

RISK FOR ASPIRATION
(1988)

Definition *At risk for entry of gastrointestinal secretions, oropharyngeal secretions, solids, or fluids into tracheobronchial passages*

Risk Factors

Increased intragastric pressure

Tube feedings

Situations hindering elevation of upper body

Reduced level of consciousness

Presence of tracheostomy or endotracheal tube

Medication administration

Wired jaws

Increased gastric residual

Incompetent lower esophageal sphincter

Impaired swallowing

Gastrointestinal tubes

Facial, oral, neck surgery or trauma

Depressed cough and gag reflexes

Decreased gastrointestinal motility

Delayed gastric emptying

RISK FOR IMPAIRED PARENT/INFANT/ CHILD **ATTACHMENT**
(1994)

Definition   *Disruption of the interactive process between parent/significant other, child, and infant that fosters the development of a protective and nurturing reciprocal relationship*

Risk Factors

Physical barriers
Anxiety associated with
    the parent role
Substance abuse
Premature infant, ill
    infant/child who is
    unable to effectively
    initiate parental contact
    due to altered behav-
    ioral organization

Lack of privacy
Inability of parents to
    meet personal needs
Separation

AUTONOMIC DYSREFLEXIA
(1988)

Definition   *Life-threatening, uninhibited sympathetic response of the nervous system to a noxious stimulus after a spinal cord injury at T7 or above*

Defining Characteristics

- Pallor (below the injury)
- Paroxysmal hypertension (sudden periodic elevated blood pressure with systolic pressure >140 mm Hg and diastolic pressure >90 mm Hg)
- Red splotches on skin (above the injury)
- Bradycardia or tachycardia (heart rate <60 or >100 beats per minute)
- Diaphoresis (above the injury)
- Headache (a diffuse pain in different portions of the head and not confined to any nerve distribution area)
- Blurred vision
- Chest pain
- Chilling
- Conjunctival congestion
- Horner's syndrome (contraction of the pupil, partial ptosis of the eyelid, enophthalmos and sometimes loss of sweating over the affected side of the face)
- Metallic taste in mouth
- Nasal congestion
- Paresthesia
- Pilomotor reflex (gooseflesh formation when skin is cooled)

Related Factors

Bladder distention
Bowel distention
Lack of patient and
    caregiver knowledge
Skin irritation

RISK FOR AUTONOMIC DYSREFLEXIA
(1998, 2000)

Definition *At risk for life-threatening, uninhibited response of the sympathetic nervous system, post spinal shock, in an individual with spinal cord injury or lesion at T6 or above (has been demonstrated in patients with injuries at T7 and T8)*

Risk Factors

An injury/lesion at T6 or above AND at least one of the following noxious stimuli:

Neurological Stimuli
- Painful/irritating stimuli below level of injury

Urological Stimuli
- Bladder distention
- Detrusor sphincter dyssynergia
- Bladder spasm
- Instrumentation or surgery
- Epididymitis
- Urethritis
- Urinary tract infection
- Calculi
- Cystitis
- Catheterization

Gastrointestinal Stimuli
- Bowel distention
- Fecal impaction
- Digital stimulation
- Suppositories
- Hemorrhoids
- Difficult passage of feces
- Constipation

- Enemas
- GI system pathology
- Gastric ulcers
- Esophageal reflux
- Gallstones

Reproductive Stimuli
- Menstruation
- Sexual intercourse
- Pregnancy
- Labor and delivery
- Ovarian cyst
- Ejaculation

Musculoskeletal-Integumentary Stimuli
- Cutaneous stimulation (e.g., pressure ulcer, ingrown toenail, dressings, burns, rash)
- Pressure over bony prominences or genitalia
- Heterotrophic bone
- Spasm
- Fractures
- Range-of-motion exercises

- Wounds
- Sunburns

Regulatory Stimuli

- Temperature fluctuations
- Extreme environmental temperatures

Situational Stimuli

- Positioning
- Constrictive clothing (e.g., straps, stockings, shoes)

- Drug reactions (e.g., decongestants, sympathomimetics, vasoconstrictors, narcotic withdrawal)
- Surgical procedure

Cardiac/Pulmonary Problems

- Pulmonary emboli
- Deep vein thrombosis

DISTURBED **B**ODY IMAGE
(1973, 1998)

Definition *Confusion in mental picture of one's physical self*

Defining Characteristics

- Verbalization of feelings that reflect an altered view of one's body in appearance, structure, or function
- Verbalization of perceptions that reflect an altered view of one's body in appearance, structure, or function
- Nonverbal response to actual or perceived change in body structure and/or function
- Behaviors of avoidance, monitoring, or acknowledgment of one's body

Objective

- Missing body part
- Trauma to nonfunctioning part
- Not touching body part
- Hiding or overexposing body part (intentional or unintentional)

- Actual change in structure and/or function
- Change in social involvement
- Change in ability to estimate spatial relationship of body to environment
- Extension of body boundary to incorporate environmental objects
- Not looking at body part

Subjective

- Refusal to verify actual change
- Preoccupation with change or loss
- Personalization of part or loss by name
- Depersonalization of part or loss by impersonal pronouns
- Extension of body boundary to incorporate environmental objects

B

- Negative feelings about body (e.g., feelings of helplessness, hopelessness, or powerlessness)
- Verbalization of change in lifestyle
- Focus on past strength, function, or appearance

- Fear of rejection or of reaction by others
- Emphasis on remaining strengths
- Heightened achievement

Related Factors

Psychosocial
Biophysical
Cognitive / perceptual
Cultural or spiritual
Developmental changes

Illness
Trauma or injury
Surgery
Illness treatment

B

RISK FOR IMBALANCED BODY TEMPERATURE
(1986, 2000)

Definition   *At risk for failure to maintain body temperature within normal range*

Risk Factors

Altered metabolic rate

Illness or trauma affecting temperature regulation

Medications causing vasoconstriction or vasodilation

Inappropriate clothing for environmental temperature

Inactivity or vigorous activity

Extremes of weight

Extremes of age

Dehydration

Sedation

Exposure to cold/cool or warm/hot environments

Bowel Incontinence
(1975, 1998)

Definition *Change in normal bowel habits characterized by involuntary passage of stool*

Defining Characteristics

- Constant dribbling of soft stool
- Fecal odor
- Inability to delay defecation
- Urgency
- Self-report of inability to feel rectal fullness
- Fecal staining of clothing and/or bedding

- Recognizes rectal fullness but reports inability to expel formed stool
- Inattention to urge to defecate
- Inability to recognize urge to defecate
- Red perianal skin

Related Factors

Environmental factors (e.g., inaccessible bathroom)

Incomplete emptying of bowel

Rectal sphincter abnormality

Impaction

Dietary habits

Colorectal lesions

Stress

Lower motor nerve damage

Abnormally high abdominal or intestinal pressure

General decline in muscle tone

Loss of rectal sphincter control

Impaired cognition

Upper motor nerve damage

Chronic diarrhea

Toileting self-care deficit

Impaired reservoir capacity

Medications

Immobility

Laxative abuse

EFFECTIVE BREASTFEEDING
(1990)

Definition *Mother-infant dyad/family exhibits adequate proficiency and satisfaction with breastfeeding process*

Defining Characteristics

- Effective mother/infant communication patterns
- Regular and sustained suckling/swallowing at the breast
- Appropriate infant weight pattern for age
- Infant content after feeding
- Mother able to position infant at breast to promote a successful latch-on response
- Signs and/or symptoms of oxytocin release
- Adequate infant elimination patterns for age
- Eagerness of infant to nurse
- Maternal verbalization of satisfaction with the breastfeeding process

Related Factors

Infant gestational age
>34 weeks
Support source
Normal infant oral
structure
Maternal confidence
Basic breastfeeding
knowledge
Normal breast structure

INEFFECTIVE BREASTFEEDING
(1988)

Definition *Dissatisfaction or difficulty a mother, infant, or child experiences with the breastfeeding process*

Defining Characteristics

- Unsatisfactory breast-feeding process
- Nonsustained suckling at the breast
- Resisting latching on
- Unresponsive to comfort measures
- Persistence of sore nipples beyond first week of breastfeeding
- Observable signs of inadequate infant intake
- Insufficient emptying of each breast per feeding
- Infant inability to attach on to maternal breast correctly
- Infant arching and crying at the breast
- Infant exhibiting fussiness and crying within the first hour after breastfeeding
- Actual or perceived inadequate milk supply
- No observable signs of oxytocin release
- Insufficient opportunity for suckling at the breast

Related Factors

Nonsupportive partner/ family
Previous breast surgery
Infant receiving supplemental feedings with artificial nipple
Prematurity
Previous history of breastfeeding failure
Poor infant sucking reflex
Maternal breast anomaly
Maternal anxiety or ambivalence
Interruption in breastfeeding
Infant anomaly
Knowledge deficit

B

INTERRUPTED BREASTFEEDING
(1992)

Definition *Break in the continuity of the breastfeeding process as a result of inability or inadvisability to put baby to breast for feeding*

Defining Characteristics

- Infant receives no nourishment at the breast for some or all of feedings
- Maternal desire to maintain and provide (or eventually provide) her breast milk for her infant's nutritional needs
- Lack of knowledge regarding expression and storage of breast milk
- Separation of mother and infant

Related Factors

Contraindications to
    breastfeeding
Maternal employment
Maternal or infant illness
Need to abruptly wean
    infant
Prematurity

INEFFECTIVE BREATHING PATTERN
(1980, 1996, 1998)

Definition *Inspiration and/or expiration that does not provide adequate ventilation*

Defining Characteristics

- Decreased inspiratory/ expiratory pressure
- Decreased minute ventilation
- Use of accessory muscles to breathe
- Nasal flaring
- Dyspnea
- Orthopnea
- Altered chest excursion
- Shortness of breath
- Assumption of 3-point position
- Pursed-lip breathing
- Prolonged expiration phases
- Increased anterior-posterior diameter
- Respiratory rate/min:
  - Infants: <25 or >60
  - Ages 1–4: <20 or >30
  - Ages 5–14: <14 or >25
  - Adults >14: ≤11 or >24
- Depth of breathing
  - Adult tidal volume: 500 ml at rest
  - Infant tidal volume: 6–8 ml/Kg
- Timing ratio
- Decreased vital capacity

Related Factors

Hyperventilation
Hypoventilation syndrome
Bony deformity
Pain
Chest wall deformity
Anxiety
Decreased energy/ fatigue
Neuromuscular dysfunction

Musculoskeletal impairment
Perception/cognitive impairment
Obesity
Spinal cord injury
Body position
Neurological immaturity
Respiratory muscle fatigue

C **C**

DECREASED Cardiac OUTPUT
(1975, 1996, 2000)

Definition *Inadequate blood pumped by the heart to meet metabolic demands of the body*

Defining Characteristics

Altered Heart Rate/ Rhythm

- Arrhythmias (tachycardia, bradycardia)
- Palpitations
- EKG changes

Altered Preload

- Jugular vein distention
- Fatigue
- Edema
- Murmurs
- Increased/decreased central venous pressure (CVP)
- Increased/decreased pulmonary artery wedge pressure (PAWP)
- Weight gain

Altered Afterload

- Cold/clammy skin
- Shortness of breath/ dyspnea
- Oliguria
- Prolonged capillary refill
- Decreased peripheral pulses

- Variations in blood pressure readings
- Increased/decreased systemic vascular resistance (SVR)
- Increased/decreased pulmonary vascular resistance (PVR)
- Skin color changes

Altered Contractility

- Crackles
- Cough
- Orthopnea/paroxysmal nocturnal dyspnea
- Cardiac output <4 L/min
- Cardiac index <2.5 L/min
- Decreased ejection fraction, Stroke Volume Index (SVI), Left Ventricular Stroke Work Index (LVSWI)
- S3 or S4 sounds

Behavioral/Emotional

- Anxiety
- Restlessness

Related Factors

Altered heart rate/
rhythm

Altered Stroke Volume

Altered preload
Altered afterload
Altered contractility

C CAREGIVER ROLE STRAIN
(1992, 1998, 2000)

Definition *Difficulty in performing family caregiver role*

Defining Characteristics

Caregiving Activities

- Difficulty performing/completing required tasks
- Preoccupation with care routine
- Apprehension about the future regarding care receiver's health and the caregiver's ability to provide care
- Apprehension about care receiver's care if caregiver becomes ill or dies
- Dysfunctional change in caregiving activities
- Apprehension about possible institutionalization of care receiver

Caregiver Health Status

Physical

- GI upset (e.g., mild stomach cramps, vomiting, diarrhea, recurrent gastric ulcer episodes)
- Weight change
- Rash
- Hypertension
- Cardiovascular disease
- Diabetes
- Fatigue
- Headaches

Emotional

- Impaired individual coping
- Feeling depressed
- Disturbed sleep
- Anger
- Stress
- Somatization
- Increased nervousness
- Increased emotional lability
- Impatience
- Lack of time to meet personal needs
- Frustration

Socioeconomic

- Withdraws from social life
- Changes in leisure activities
- Low work productivity
- Refuses career advancement

C

Caregiver-Care Receiver Relationship

- Grief/uncertainty regarding changed relationship with care receiver
- Difficulty watching care receiver go through the illness

Family Processes

- Family conflict
- Concerns about family members

Related Factors

Care Receiver Health Status

Illness severity
Illness chronicity
Increasing care needs/ dependency
Unpredictability of illness course
Instability of care receiver's health
Problem behaviors
Psychological or cognitive problems
Addiction or codependency

Caregiving Activities

Amount of activities
Complexity of activities
24-hour care responsibilities
Ongoing changes in activities
Discharge of family members to home with significant care needs

Years of caregiving
Unpredictability of care situation

Caregiver Health Status

Physical problems
Psychological or cognitive problems
Addiction or codependency
Marginal coping patterns
Unrealistic expectations of self
Inability to fulfill one's own or other's expectations

Socioeconomic

Isolation from others
Competing role commitments
Alienation from family, friends, and co-workers
Insufficient recreation

continued

Caregiver Role Strain, *continued*

C

Caregiver-Care Receiver Relationship

History of poor relationship

Presence of abuse or violence

Unrealistic expectations of caregiver by care receiver

Mental status of elder inhibiting conversation

Family Processes

History of marginal family coping

History of family dysfunction

Resources

Inadequate physical environment for providing care (e.g., housing, temperature, safety)

Inadequate equipment for providing care

Inadequate transportation

Inadequate community resources (e.g., respite services, recreational resources)

Insufficient finances

Lack of support

Caregiver is not developmentally ready for caregiver role

Inexperience with caregiving

Insufficient time

Lack of knowledge about or difficulty accessing community resources

Lack of caregiver privacy

Emotional strength

Physical energy

Assistance and support (formal and informal)

RISK FOR Caregiver role strain

(1992)

C

Definition *Caregiver is vulnerable for felt difficulty in performing the family caregiver role*

Risk Factors

Caregiver not developmentally ready for caregiver role (e.g., a young adult needing to provide care for a middle-aged person)

Inadequate physical environment for providing care (e.g., housing, transportation, community services, equipment)

Unpredictable illness course or instability in the care receiver's health

Psychological or cognitive problems in care receiver

Presence of situational stressors that normally affect families (e.g., significant loss, disaster or crisis, economic vulnerability, major life events)

Presence of abuse or violence

Premature birth/congenital defect

Past history of poor relationship between caregiver and care receiver

Marginal family adaptation or dysfunction prior to the caregiving situation

Marginal caregiver's coping patterns

Lack of respite and recreation for caregiver

Inexperience with caregiving

Caregiver is female

Addiction or codependency

Care receiver exhibits deviant, bizarre behavior

Caregiver's competing role commitments

Caregiver health impairment

Illness severity of the care receiver

Caregiver is spouse

Developmental delay or retardation of the care receiver or caregiver

continued

Risk for Caregiver Role Strain, *continued*

C

Complexity / amount of
  caregiving tasks
Discharge of family
  member with significant
  home care needs
Duration of caregiving
  required
Family / caregiver isolation

IMPAIRED VERBAL COMMUNICATION
(1983, 1996, 1998)

Definition *Decreased, delayed, or absent ability to receive, process, transmit, and use a system of symbols*

Defining Characteristics

- Willful refusal to speak
- Disorientation in the three spheres of time, space, person
- Inability to speak dominant language
- Does not or cannot speak
- Speaks or verbalizes with difficulty
- Inappropriate verbalization
- Difficulty forming words or sentences (e.g., aphonia, dyslalia, dysarthria)
- Difficulty expressing thought verbally (e.g., aphasia, dysphasia, apraxia, dyslexia)
- Stuttering
- Slurring
- Dyspnea
- Absence of eye contact or difficulty in selective attending
- Difficulty in comprehending and maintaining usual communication pattern
- Partial or total visual deficit
- Inability or difficulty in use of facial or body expressions

Related Factors

Decrease in circulation to brain

Cultural differences

Psychological barriers (e.g., psychosis, lack of stimuli)

Physical barrier (e.g., tracheostomy, intubation)

Anatomical defect (e.g., cleft palate, alteration of the neuromuscular visual system, auditory system, phonatory apparatus)

Brain tumor

Differences related to developmental age

continued

Impaired Verbal Communication, *continued*

C

Side effects of medication
Environmental barriers
Absence of significant
  others
Altered perceptions
Lack of information
Stress
Alteration of self-esteem
  or self-concept

Physiological conditions
Alteration of central
  nervous system
Weakening of the muscu-
  loskeletal system
Emotional conditions

READINESS FOR ENHANCED COMMUNICATION
(2002, LOE 2.1)

Definition *A pattern of exchanging information and ideas with others that is sufficient for meeting one's needs and life's goals and can be strengthened.*

Defining Characteristics

- Expresses willingness to enhance communication
- Able to speak or write a language
- Forms words, phrases, and language
- Expresses thoughts and feelings
- Uses and interprets non-verbal cues appropriately
- Expresses satisfaction with ability to share information and ideas with others

References

Forchuck, C., Westwell, J., Martin, M., Bamber-Azzapardi, W., Kosterewa-Tolman, D., & Hux, M. (2000). The developing nurse-client relationship: Nurses' perspectives. *Journal of the American Psychiatric Nurses Association, 6,* 3–10.

Gilbert, D.A. (1998). Relational message themes in nurses' listening behavior during brief patient-nurse interactions. *Scholarly Inquiry for Nursing Practice, 12,* 5–21.

Riegel, B., Moser, D., Daugherty, J., Sornborger, K., & Saarmann, L. (2002). Can we talk? Developing a social support nursing intervention for couples. *Clinical Nurse Specialist: The Journal for Advanced Nursing Practice, 16,* 211–218.

C DECISIONAL CONFLICT (Specify)
(1988)

Definition *Uncertainty about course of action to be taken when choice among competing actions involves risk, loss, or challenge to personal life values*

Defining Characteristics

- Verbalizes uncertainty about choices
- Verbalizes undesired consequences of alternative actions being considered
- Vacillation among alternative choices
- Delayed decision making
- Verbalizes feeling of distress while attempting a decision
- Self-focusing
- Physical signs of distress or tension (e.g., increased heart rate, increased muscle tension, restlessness)
- Questioning personal values and beliefs while attempting a decision

Related Factors

Support system deficit
Perceived threat to value system
Lack of experience or interference with decision making
Multiple or divergent sources of information
Lack of relevant information
Unclear personal values/ beliefs

PARENTAL ROLE **C**ONFLICT
(1988)

C

Definition *Parent experience of role confusion and conflict in response to crisis*

Defining Characteristics

- Parent(s) express(es) concern(s) about changes in parental role, family functioning, family communication, family health
- Parent(s) express(es) concern(s)/feeling(s) of inadequacy to provide for child's physical and emotional needs during hospitalization or in home
- Reluctant to participate in usual caretaking activities even with encouragement and support
- Demonstrated disruption in caretaking routines
- Expresses concern about perceived loss of control over decisions relating to their child
- Verbalizes or demonstrates feelings of guilt, anger, fear, anxiety, and/or frustrations about effect of child's illness on family process

Related Factors

Change in marital status
Home care of a child with special needs (e.g., apnea monitoring, postural drainage, hyperalimentation)
Interruptions of family life due to home care regimen (e.g., treatments, caregivers, lack of respite)
Specialized care-center policies
Separation from child due to chronic illness
Intimidation with invasive or restrictive modalities (e.g., isolation, intubation)

C

ACUTE CONFUSION
(1994)

Definition *Abrupt onset of a cluster of global, transient changes and disturbances in attention, cognition, psychomotor activity, level of consciousness, and/or sleep/wake cycle*

Defining Characteristics

- Lack of motivation to initiate and/or follow through with goal-directed or purposeful behavior
- Fluctuation in psychomotor activity
- Misperceptions
- Fluctuation in cognition
- Increased agitation or restlessness
- Fluctuation in level of consciousness
- Fluctuation in sleep-wake cycle
- Hallucinations

Related Factors

Over 60 years of age
Alcohol abuse
Delirium
Dementia
Drug abuse

CHRONIC CONFUSION
(1994)

C

Definition *Irreversible, long-standing, and/or progressive deterioration of intellect and personality characterized by decreased ability to interpret environmental stimuli; decreased capacity for intellectual thought processes; and manifested by disturbances of memory, orientation, and behavior*

Defining Characteristics

- Altered interpretation/ response to stimuli
- Clinical evidence of organic impairment
- Progressive/long-standing cognitive impairment
- Altered personality
- Impaired memory (short- and long-term)
- Impaired socialization
- No change in level of consciousness

Related Factors

Multi-infarct dementia
Korsakoff's psychosis
Head injury
Alzheimer's disease
Cerebral vascular accident

C

CONSTIPATION
(1975, 1998)

Definition *Decrease in normal frequency of defecation accompanied by difficult or incomplete passage of stool and/or passage of excessively hard, dry stool*

Defining Characteristics

- Change in bowel pattern
- Bright red blood with stool
- Presence of soft, pastelike stool in rectum
- Distended abdomen
- Dark, black, or tarry stool
- Increased abdominal pressure
- Percussed abdominal dullness
- Pain with defecation
- Decreased volume of stool
- Straining with defecation
- Decreased frequency
- Dry, hard, formed stool
- Palpable rectal mass
- Feeling of rectal fullness or pressure
- Abdominal pain
- Unable to pass stool
- Anorexia
- Headache
- Change in abdominal growling (borborygmi)
- Indigestion
- Atypical presentations in older adults (e.g., change in mental status, urinary incontinence, unexplained falls, elevated body temperature)
- Severe flatus
- Generalized fatigue
- Hypoactive or hyperactive bowel sounds
- Palpable abdominal mass
- Abdominal tenderness with or without palpable muscle resistance
- Nausea and/or vomiting
- Oozing liquid stool

Related Factors

Functional

Recent environmental changes

Habitual denial/ignoring of urge to defecate

Insufficient physical activity

Irregular defecation habits

Inadequate toileting (e.g., timeliness, positioning for defecation, privacy)

Abdominal muscle weakness

Psychological

Depression

Emotional stress

Mental confusion

Pharmacological

Anticonvulsants

Antilipemic agents

Laxative overdose

Calcium carbonate

Aluminum-containing antacids

Nonsteroidal anti-inflammatory agents

Opiates

Anticholinergics

Diuretics

Iron salts

Phenothiazines

Sedatives

Sympathomimetics

Bismuth salts

Antidepressants

Calcium channel blockers

Mechanical

Rectal abscess or ulcer

Pregnancy

Rectal anal fissures

Tumors

Megacolon (Hirschsprung's disease)

Electrolyte imbalance

Rectal prolapse

Prostate enlargement

Neurological impairment

Rectal anal stricture

Rectocele

Postsurgical obstruction

Hemorrhoids

Obesity

Physiological

Poor eating habits

Decreased motility of gastrointestinal tract

Inadequate dentition or oral hygiene

Insufficient fiber intake

Insufficient fluid intake

Change in usual foods and eating patterns

Dehydration

C

PERCEIVED CONSTIPATION
(1988)

Definition   *Self-diagnosis of constipation and abuse of laxatives, enemas, and suppositories to ensure a daily bowel movement*

Defining Characteristics

- Expectation of a daily bowel movement with resulting overuse of laxatives, enemas, and suppositories
- Expectation of passage of stool at same time every day

Related Factors

Impaired thought processes
Faulty appraisal
Cultural/family health beliefs

RISK FOR CONSTIPATION
(1998)

C

Definition *At risk for a decrease in normal frequency of defecation accompanied by difficult or incomplete passage of stool and/or passage of excessively hard, dry stool*

Risk Factors

Functional

Habitual denial/ignoring of urge to defecate

Recent environmental changes

Inadequate toileting (e.g., timeliness, positioning for defecation, privacy)

Irregular defecation habits

Insufficient physical activity

Abdominal muscle weakness

Psychological

Emotional stress

Mental confusion

Depression

Physiological

Insufficient fiber intake

Dehydration

Inadequate dentition or oral hygiene

Poor eating habits

Insufficient fluid intake

Change in usual foods and eating patterns

Decreased motility of gastrointestinal tract

Pharmacological

Anticonvulsants

Phenothiazines

Nonsteroidal anti-inflammatory agents

Sedatives

Aluminum-containing antacids

Laxative overuse

Iron salts

Anticholinergics

Antidepressants

Antilipemic agents

Calcium channel blockers

Calcium carbonate

Diuretics

Sympathomimetics

Opiates

Bismuth salts

Mechanical

Rectal abscess or ulcer

Pregnancy

Rectal anal stricture

Postsurgical obstruction

Rectal anal fissures

Megacolon (Hirschsprung's disease)

continued

Risk for Constipation, *continued*

C

Electrolyte imbalance
Tumors
Prostate enlargement
Rectocele
Rectal prolapse
Neurological impairment
Hemorrhoids
Obesity

INEFFECTIVE COPING
(1978, 1998)

Definition *Inability to form a valid appraisal of the stressors, inadequate choices of practiced responses, and/or inability to use available resources*

Defining Characteristics

- Lack of goal-directed behavior/resolution of problem, including inability to attend to and difficulty organizing information
- Sleep disturbance
- Abuse of chemical agents
- Decreased use of social support
- Use of forms of coping that impede adaptive behavior
- Poor concentration
- Fatigue
- Inadequate problem solving
- Verbalization of inability to cope or inability to ask for help
- Inability to meet basic needs
- Destructive behavior toward self or others
- Inability to meet role expectations
- High illness rate
- Change in usual communication patterns
- Risk taking

Related Factors

Gender differences in coping strategies
Inadequate level of confidence in ability to cope
Uncertainty
Inadequate social support created by characteristics of relationships
Inadequate level of perception of control
Inadequate resources available

High degree of threat
Situational or maturational crisis
Disturbance in pattern of tension release
Inadequate opportunity to prepare for stressor
Inability to conserve adaptive energies
Disturbance in pattern of appraisal of threat

C DEFENSIVE COPING
(1988)

Definition *Repeated projection of falsely positive self-evaluation based on a self-protective pattern that defends against underlying perceived threats to positive self-regard*

Defining Characteristics

- Grandiosity
- Rationalization of failures
- Hypersensitivity to slight/criticism
- Denial of obvious problems/weaknesses
- Projection of blame/responsibility
- Lack of follow-through or participation in treatment or therapy
- Superior attitude toward others
- Hostile laughter or ridicule of others
- Difficulty in perception of reality/reality testing
- Difficulty establishing/maintaining relationships

Related Factors

To be developed

READINESS FOR ENHANCED COPING
(2002, LOE 2.1)

C

Definition *A pattern of cognitive and behavioral efforts to manage demands that is sufficient for well-being and can be strengthened.*

Defining Characteristics
- Defines stressors as manageable
- Seeks social support
- Uses a broad range of problem-oriented and emotion-oriented strategies
- Uses spiritual resources
- Acknowledges power
- Seeks knowledge of new strategies
- Is aware of possible environmental changes

References

Fredrickson, B.L., & Joiner, T. (2002). Positive emotions trigger upward spirals toward emotional well-being. *Psychological Science: A Journal of the American Psychological Association, 13*(2), 172–175.

Pender, N.J., Murdaugh, C.L., & Parsons, M.A. (2002). Stress management and health [Chapter 10]; Social support and health [Chapter 11]. In *Health promotion in nursing practice* (4th ed., pp. 217–255). Upper Saddle River, NJ: Prentice Hall.

Rahe, R.H., Taylor, C.B., Tolles, R.L., Newall, L.M., Veach, T.L., & Bryson, S. (2002). A novel stress and coping workplace program reduces illness and healthcare utilization. *Psychosomatic Medicine, 64*(2), 278–286.

C

INEFFECTIVE COMMUNITY COPING
(1994, 1998)

Definition *Pattern of community activities (for adaptation and problem solving) that is unsatisfactory for meeting the demands or needs of the community*

Defining Characteristics

- Expressed community powerlessness
- Deficits in community participation
- Excessive community conflicts
- Expressed vulnerability
- High illness rates
- Stressors perceived as excessive

- Community does not meet its own expectations
- Increased social problems (e.g., homicides, vandalism, arson, terrorism, robbery, infanticide, abuse, divorce, unemployment, poverty, militancy, mental illness)

Related Factors

Natural or man-made disasters

Ineffective or nonexistent community systems (e.g., lack of emergency medical system, transportation system, or disaster planning systems)

Deficits in community social support services and resources

Inadequate resources for problem solving

READINESS FOR ENHANCED COMMUNITY COPING

(1994)

Definition *Pattern of community activities for adaptation and problem solving that is satisfactory for meeting the demands or needs of the community but can be improved for management of current and future problems/stressors*

Defining Characteristics

- One or more characteristics that indicate effective coping:
  - Positive communication between community/aggregates and larger community
  - Programs available for recreation and relaxation
  - Resources sufficient for managing stressors
  - Agreement that community is responsible for stress management
  - Active planning by community for predicted stressors
  - Active problem solving by community when faced with issues
  - Positive communication among community members

Related Factors

Community has a sense of power to manage stressors
Social supports available
Resources available for problem solving

C

COMPROMISED FAMILY COPING
(1980, 1996)

Definition   *Usually supportive primary person (family member or close friend) provides insufficient, ineffective, or compromised support, comfort, assistance, or encouragement that may be needed by the client to manage or master adaptive tasks related to his/her health challenge*

Defining Characteristics

Objective

- Significant person attempts assistive or supportive behaviors with less than satisfactory results
- Significant person displays protective behavior disproportionate (too little or too much) to client's abilities or need for autonomy
- Significant person withdraws or enters into limited or temporary personal communication with client at the time of need

Subjective

- Client expresses or confirms a concern or complaint about significant other's response to his/her health problem
- Significant person describes or confirms an inadequate understanding or knowledge base, which interferes with effective assistive or supportive behaviors
- Significant person describes preoccupation with personal reaction (e.g., fear, anticipatory grief, guilt, anxiety) to client's illness, disability, or other situational or developmental crisis

Related Factors

Temporary preoccupation by a significant person who tries to manage emotional conflicts and personal suffering and is unable to perceive or act effectively in regard to client's needs

Temporary family disorganization and role changes

Prolonged disease or progression of disability that exhausts supportive capacity of significant people

Other situational or developmental crises or situations the significant person may be facing

Inadequate or incorrect information or understanding by a primary person

Little support provided by client, in turn, for primary person

C

DISABLED FAMILY COPING
(1980, 1996)

Definition *Behavior of significant person (family member or other primary person) that disables his/her capacities and the client's capacities to effectively address tasks essential to either person's adaption to the health challenge*

Defining Characteristics

- Intolerance
- Agitation, depression, aggression, hostility
- Taking on illness signs of client
- Rejection
- Psychosomaticism
- Neglectful relationships with other family members
- Neglectful care of client in regard to basic human needs and/or illness treatment
- Distortion of reality regarding client's health problem, including extreme denial about its existence or severity
- Impaired restructuring of a meaningful life for self
- Impaired individualization, prolonged overconcern for client
- Desertion
- Decisions and actions by family that are detrimental to economic or social well-being
- Carrying on usual routines, disregarding client's needs
- Abandonment
- Client's development of helpless, inactive dependence
- Disregarding needs

Related Factors

Significant person with chronically unexpressed feelings of quilt, anxiety, hostility, despair, etc.

Arbitrary handling of family's resistance to treatment, which tends to solidify defensiveness as it fails to deal adequately with underlying anxiety

Dissonant or discrepant coping styles for dealing with adaptive tasks by the significant person and client or among significant people

Highly ambivalent family relationships

C   READINESS FOR ENHANCED FAMILY COPING
(1980)

Definition   *Effective management of adaptive tasks by family member involved with the client's health challenge, who now exhibits desire and readiness for enhanced health and growth in regard to self and in relation to the client*

Defining Characteristics

- Individual expresses interest in making contact on a one-to-one basis or on a mutual-aid group basis with another person who has experienced a similar situation
- Family member attempts to describe growth impact of crisis on his/ her own values, priorities, goal, or relationships
- Family member moves in direction of health-promoting and enriching life-style that supports and monitors maturational processes, audits and negotiates treatment programs, and chooses experiences that optimize wellness

Related Factors

Needs sufficiently gratified and adaptive tasks effectively addressed to enable goals of self-actualization to surface

RISK FOR SUDDEN INFANT **D**EATH SYNDROME
(2002, LOE 3.3)

Definition *Presence of risk factors for sudden death of an infant under 1 year of age*

Risk Factors

Modifiable

Infants placed to sleep in the prone or side-lying position

Prenatal and/or post-natal infant smoke exposure

Infant overheating/overwrapping

Soft underlayment/loose articles in the sleep environment

Delayed or nonattendance of prenatal care

Potentially Modifiable

Low birth weight

Prematurity

Young maternal age

Nonmodifiable

Male gender

Ethnicity (e.g., African American or Native American race of mother)

Seasonality of SIDS deaths (higher in winter and fall months)

SIDS mortality peaks between infant age of 2–4 months

continued

Risk for Sudden Infant Death Syndrome, *continued*

References

American Academy of Pediatrics, Task Force on Infant Sleep Position and Sudden Infant Death Syndrome. (2000). Changing concepts of sudden infant death syndrome: Implications for infant sleeping environment and sleep position (RE9946). *Pediatrics, 105,* 650–656.

Heln, H.A., & S.F. Pettit. (2001). Back to sleep: Good advice for parents but not for hospitals? *Pediatrics, 107,* 537–539.

Willinger, M., James, L., & Catz, C. (1991). Defining the sudden infant death syndrome (SIDS): Deliberations of an expert panel convened by the National Institute of Child Health and Human Development. *Pediatric Pathology, 11,* 677–684.

INEFFECTIVE DENIAL
(1988)

Definition *Conscious or unconscious attempt to disavow the knowledge or meaning of an event to reduce anxiety/fear, but leading to the detriment of health*

Defining Characteristics

- Delays seeking or refuses healthcare attention to the detriment of health
- Does not perceive personal relevance of symptoms or danger
- Displaces source of symptoms to other organs
- Displays inappropriate affect
- Does not admit fear of death or invalidism
- Makes dismissive gestures or comments when speaking of distressing events
- Minimizes symptoms
- Unable to admit impact of disease on life pattern
- Uses home remedies (self-treatment) to relieve symptoms
- Displaces fear of impact of the condition

Related Factors

To be developed

D

IMPAIRED DENTITION
(1998)

Definition *Disruption in tooth development/eruption patterns or structural integrity of individual teeth*

Defining Characteristics

- Excessive plaque
- Crown or root caries
- Halitosis
- Tooth enamel discoloration
- Toothache
- Loose teeth
- Excessive calculus
- Incomplete eruption for age (may be primary or permanent teeth)
- Malocclusion or tooth misalignment
- Premature loss of primary teeth
- Worn down or abraded teeth
- Tooth fracture(s)
- Missing teeth or complete absence
- Erosion of enamel
- Asymmetrical facial expression

Related Factors

Ineffective oral hygiene, sensitivity to heat or cold
Barriers to self-care
Access or economic barriers to professional care
Nutritional deficits
Dietary habits
Genetic predisposition
Selected prescription medications
Premature loss of primary teeth
Excessive intake of fluorides
Chronic vomiting
Chronic use of tobacco, coffee or tea, red wine
Lack of knowledge regarding dental health
Excessive use of abrasive cleaning agents
Bruxism

RISK FOR DELAYED DEVELOPMENT
(1998)

D

Definition   *At risk for delay of 25% or more in one or more of the areas of social or self-regulatory behavior, or in cognitive, language, gross or fine motor skills*

Risk Factors

Prenatal

Maternal age <15 or >35 years
Substance abuse
Infections
Genetic or endocrine disorders
Unplanned or unwanted pregnancy
Lack of, late, or poor prenatal care
Inadequate nutrition
Illiteracy
Poverty

Individual

Prematurity
Seizures
Congenital or genetic disorders
Positive drug screening test
Brain damage (e.g., hemorrhage in postnatal period, shaken baby, abuse, accident)

Vision impairment
Hearing impairment or frequent otitis media
Chronic illness
Technology-dependent
Failure to thrive, inadequate nutrition
Foster or adopted child
Lead poisoning
Chemotherapy
Radiation therapy
Natural disaster
Behavior disorders
Substance abuse

Environmental

Poverty
Violence

Caregiver

Abuse
Mental illness
Mental retardation or severe learning disability

Diarrhea
(1975, 1998)

Definition   *Passage of loose, unformed stools*

Defining Characteristics

- At least 3 loose liquid stools per day
- Hyperactive bowel sounds
- Urgency
- Abdominal pain
- Cramping

Related Factors

Psychological

High stress levels and anxiety

Situational

Alcohol abuse
Toxins
Laxative abuse
Radiation
Tube feedings
Adverse effects of medications
Contaminants
Travel

Physiological

Inflammation
Malabsorption
Infectious processes
Irritation
Parasites

RISK FOR Disuse SYNDROME
(1988)

Definition *At risk for deterioration of body systems as the result of prescribed or unavoidable musculoskeletal inactivity*

Risk Factors
Severe pain
Mechanical
  immobilization
Altered level of
  consciousness
Prescribed immobilization
Paralysis

Note. Complications from immobility can include pressure ulcer, constipation, stasis of pulmonary secretions, thrombosis, urinary tract infection and / or retention, decreased strength or endurance, orthostatic hypotension, decreased range of joint motion, disorientation, body-image disturbance, and powerlessness.

DEFICIENT DIVERSIONAL ACTIVITY
(1980)

D

Definition *Decreased stimulation from (or interest or engagement in) recreational or leisure activities*

Defining Characteristics
- Usual hobbies cannot be undertaken in hospital
- Patient's statements regarding: boredom, wish there was something to do, to read, etc.

Related Factors

Environmental lack of diversional activity as in long-term hospitalization, frequent lengthy treatments

DISTURBED Energy Field
(1994, 2004, LOE 2.1)

E

Definition *Disruption of the flow of energy surrounding a person's being results in disharmony of the body, mind, and/or spirit*

Defining Characteristics

- Perceptions of changes in patterns of energy flow, such as
  - Movement (wave, spike, tingling, dense, flowing)
  - Sounds (tone, words)
  - Temperature change (warmth, coolness)
  - Visual changes (image, color)
  - Disruption of the field (deficit, hole, spike, bulge, obstruction, congestion, diminished flow in energy field)

Related Factors

Slowing or blocking of energy flows secondary to:

Pathophysiologic factors
  Illness (specify)
  Pregnancy
  Injury

Treatment-related factors
  Immobility
  Labor and delivery
  Perioperative experience
  Chemotherapy

Situational factors
(personal, environmental)
  Pain
  Fear
  Anxiety
  Grieving

Maturational factors
  Age-related developmental difficulties or crisis (specify)

continued

Disturbed Energy Field, *continued*

References

Macrae, J. (1988). *Therapeutic touch: A practical guide.* New York: Knopf.

Newshan, G., & Schuller-Civitella, D. (2003). Large clinical study shows value of therapeutic touch program. *Holistic Nursing Practice, 17,* 189–192.

Nurse Healers Professional Associates International, the official organization of Therapeutic Touch™. 3760 S. Highland Drive, Salt Lake City, Utah 84106; www.therapeutic-touch.org.

E

IMPAIRED ENVIRONMENTAL INTERPRETATION SYNDROME
(1994)

E

Definition *Consistent lack of orientation to person, place, time, or circumstances over more than 3 to 6 months necessitating a protective environment*

Defining Characteristics

- Consistent disorientation in known and unknown environments
- Chronic confusional states
- Loss of occupation or social functioning from memory decline
- Inability to follow simple directions, instructions
- Inability to concentrate
- Inability to reason
- Slow in responding to questions

Related Factors

Depression
Huntington's disease
Dementia (e.g.,
   Alzheimer's, multi-
   infarct, Pick's disease,
   AIDS, alcoholism,
   Parkinson's disease)

ADULT **F**AILURE TO THRIVE
(1998)

Definition *Progressive functional deterioration of a physical and cognitive nature. The individual's ability to live with multisystem diseases, cope with ensuing problems, and manage his/her care are remarkably diminished.*

Defining Characteristics

- Anorexia: Does not eat meals when offered
- States does not have an appetite, not hungry, or "I don't want to eat"
- Inadequate nutritional intake: Eating less than body requirements
- Consumption of minimal to no food at most meals (i.e., consumes <75% of normal requirements)
- Weight loss (decreased from baseline weight)
  - 5% unintentional weight loss in 1 month
  - 10% unintentional weight loss in 6 months
- Physical decline (decline in bodily function): Evidence of fatigue, dehydration, incontinence of bowel and bladder

- Frequent exacerbations of chronic health problems (e.g., pneumonia, urinary tract infections)
- Cognitive decline (decline in mental processing) as evidenced by:
  - Problems with responding appropriately to environmental stimuli
  - Demonstrated difficulty in reasoning, decision making, judgment, memory and concentration
  - Decreased perception
- Decreased social skills/social withdrawal: Noticeable decrease from usual past behavior in attempts to form or participate in cooperative and interdependent rela-

tionships (e.g., decreased verbal communication with staff, family, friends)
- Decreased participation in activities of daily living that the older person once enjoyed
- Self-care deficit: No longer looks after or takes charge of physical cleanliness or appearance
- Difficulty performing simple self-care tasks
- Neglect of home environment and/or financial responsibilities

- Apathy as evidenced by lack of observable feeling or emotion in terms of normal activities of daily living and environment
- Altered mood state: Expresses feelings of sadness, being low in spirit
- Expresses loss of interest in pleasurable outlets such as food, sex, work, friends, family, hobbies, or entertainment
- Verbalizes desire for death

Related Factors

Depression
Apathy
Fatigue

RISK FOR FALLS
(2000)

Definition *Increased susceptibility to falling that may cause physical harm*

Risk Factors

Adults

History of falls
Wheelchair use
Age 65 or over
Female (if elderly)
Lives alone
Lower limb prosthesis
Use of assistive devices
  (e.g., walker, cane)
Physiological
Presence of acute illness
Postoperative conditions
Visual difficulties
Hearing difficulties
Arthritis
Orthostatic hypotension
Sleeplessness
Faintness when turning
  or extending neck
Anemias
Vascular disease
Neoplasms (i.e.,
  fatigue/limited mobility)
Urgency and/or
  incontinence
Diarrhea
Decreased lower
  extremity strength
Postprandial blood sugar
  changes

Foot problems
Impaired physical mobility
Impaired balance
Difficulty with gait
Proprioceptive deficits
  (e.g., unilateral neglect)
Neuropathy
Cognitive
Diminished mental status
  (e.g., confusion,
  delirium, dementia,
  impaired reality testing)
Medications
Antihypertensive agents
ACE inhibitors
Diuretics
Tricyclic antidepressants
Alcohol use
Antianxiety agents
Narcotics
Hypnotics or tranquilizers
Environment
Restraints
Weather conditions (e.g.,
  wet floors/ice)
Throw/scatter rugs
Cluttered environment
Unfamiliar, dimly lit room
No antislip material in
  bath and/or shower

Children

<2 years of age
Male gender when <1
  year of age
Lack of auto restraints
Lack of gate on stairs

Lack of window guard
Bed located near window
Unattended infant on bed/
  changing table/sofa
Lack of parental
  supervision

DYSFUNCTIONAL **F**AMILY PROCESSES: ALCOHOLISM
(1994)

Definition   *Psychosocial, spiritual, and physiological functions of the family unit are chronically disorganized, which leads to conflict, denial of problems, resistance to change, ineffective problem solving, and a series of self-perpetuating crises*

Defining Characteristics
Roles and Relationships

- Inconsistent parenting/ low perception of parental support
- Ineffective spouse communication/marital problems
- Intimacy dysfunction
- Deterioration in family relationships/disturbed family dynamics
- Altered role function/ disruption of family roles
- Closed communication systems
- Chronic family problems
- Family denial
- Lack of cohesiveness
- Neglected obligations
- Lack of skills necessary for relationships
- Reduced ability of family members to relate to each other for mutual growth and maturation
- Disrupted family rituals

- Family unable to meet security needs of its members
- Economic problems
- Family does not demonstrate respect for individuality and autonomy of its members
- Triangulating family relationships
- Pattern of rejection

Behavioral

- Refusal to get help/ inability to accept and receive help appropriately
- Inadequate understanding or knowledge of alcoholism
- Ineffective problem-solving skills
- Manipulation
- Rationalization/denial of problems
- Blaming, criticizing
- Inability to meet emotional needs of its members

- Alcohol abuse
- Broken promises
- Dependency
- Impaired communication
- Difficulty with intimate relationships
- Enabling to maintain alcoholic drinking pattern
- Inappropriate expression of anger
- Isolation
- Inability to meet spiritual needs of its members
- Inability to express or accept wide range of feelings
- Inability to deal constructively with traumatic experiences
- Inability to adapt to change
- Immaturity
- Harsh self-judgment
- Lying
- Lack of dealing with conflict
- Lack of reliability
- Nicotine addiction
- Orientation toward tension relief rather than achievement of goals

- Seeking approval and affirmation
- Difficulty having fun
- Agitation
- Chaos
- Contradictory, paradoxical communication
- Diminished physical contact
- Disturbances in academic performance in children
- Disturbances in concentration
- Escalating conflict
- Failure to accomplish current or past developmental tasks / difficulty with life cycle transitions
- Family special occasions are alcohol centered
- Controlling communication / power struggles
- Self-blaming
- Stress-related physical illnesses
- Substance abuse other than alcohol
- Unresolved grief
- Verbal abuse of spouse or parent

F

continued

Dysfunctional Family Processes: Alcoholism, *continued*

Feelings

- Insecurity
- Lingering resentment
- Mistrust
- Vulnerability
- Rejection
- Repressed emotions
- Responsibility for alcoholic's behavior
- Shame/embarrassment
- Unhappiness
- Powerlessness
- Anger/suppressed rage
- Anxiety, tension, or distress
- Emotional isolation/ loneliness
- Frustration
- Guilt
- Hopelessness
- Hurt
- Decreased self-esteem/ worthlessness
- Hostility
- Lack of identity
- Fear
- Loss
- Emotional control by others
- Misunderstood
- Moodiness
- Abandonment
- Being different from other people
- Being unloved
- Confused love and pity
- Confusion
- Failure
- Depression
- Dissatisfaction

Related Factors

Abuse of alcohol
Genetic predisposition
Lack of problem-solving skills
Inadequate coping skills

Family history of alcoholism, resistance to treatment
Biochemical influences
Addictive personality

INTERRUPTED FAMILY PROCESSES
(1982, 1998)

Definition *Change in family relationships and/or functioning*

Defining Characteristics

- Changes in
  - Power alliances
  - Assigned tasks
  - Effectiveness in completing assigned tasks
  - Mutual support
  - Availability for affective responsiveness and intimacy
  - Patterns and rituals
  - Participation in problem solving
  - Participation in decision making
  - Communication patterns
  - Availability for emotional support
  - Satisfaction with family
  - Stress-reduction behaviors
  - Expressions of conflict with and/or isolation from community resources
  - Somatic complaints
  - Expressions of conflict within family

Related Factors

Power shift of family members

Family roles shift

Shift in health status of a family member

Developmental transition and/or crisis

Situation transition and/or crises

Informal or formal interaction with community

Modification in family social status

Modification in family finances

READINESS FOR ENHANCED FAMILY PROCESSES
(2002, LOE 2.1)

Definition *A pattern of family functioning that is sufficient to support the well-being of family members and can be strengthened*

Defining Characteristics

- Expresses willingness to enhance family dynamics
- Family functioning meets physical, social, and psychological needs of family members
- Activities support the safety and growth of family members
- Communication is adequate
- Relationships are generally positive; interdependent with community; family task are accomplished
- Family roles are flexible and appropriate for developmental stages
- Respect for family members is evident
- Family adapts to change
- Boundaries of family members are maintained
- Energy level of family supports activities of daily living
- Family resilience is evident
- Balance exists between autonomy and cohesiveness

References

Bryan, A.A. (2000). Enhancing parent-child interaction with a prenatal couple intervention. *The American Journal of Maternal/Child Nursing, 25*(3), 139–145.

Carruth, A.K., & Tate, U.S. (1997). Reciprocity, emotional well-being, and family functioning as determinants of family satisfaction in caregivers of elderly parents. *Nursing Research, 46*(2), 93–100.

Edelman, C.L., & Mandle, C.L. (2002). Health promotion of the family [Chapter 7]. In *Health promotion throughout the lifespan* (5th ed., pp. 169–198). St. Louis, MO: Mosby.

Fatigue
(1988, 1998)

Definition *An overwhelming sustained sense of exhaustion and decreased capacity for physical and mental work at usual level*

Defining Characteristics

- Inability to restore energy even after sleep
- Lack of energy or inability to maintain usual level of physical activity
- Increase in rest requirements
- Tired
- Verbalization of an unremitting and overwhelming lack of energy
- Inability to maintain usual routines
- Lethargic or listless
- Increase in physical complaints
- Perceived need for additional energy to accomplish routine tasks
- Compromised concentration
- Disinterest in surroundings, introspection
- Decreased performance
- Compromised libido
- Drowsy
- Feelings of guilt for not keeping up with responsibilities

Related Factors

Psychological

Boring lifestyle
Stress
Anxiety
Depression

Environmental

Humidity
Lights
Noise
Temperature

Situational

Negative life events
Occupation

Physiological

Sleep deprivation
Pregnancy
Poor physical condition
Disease states
Increased physical exertion
Malnutrition
Anemia

Fear
(1980, 1996, 2000)

Definition *Response to perceived threat that is consciously recognized as a danger*

F

Defining Characteristics

- Report of
  - Apprehension
  - Increased tension
  - Decreased self-assurance
  - Excitement
  - Being scared
  - Jitteriness
  - Dread
  - Alarm
  - Terror
  - Panic

Cognitive

- Identifies object of fear
- Stimulus believed to be a threat
- Diminished productivity, learning ability, problem-solving ability

Behaviors

- Increased alertness
- Avoidance or attack behaviors
- Impulsiveness
- Narrowed focus on "it" (i.e., the focus of the fear)

Physiological

- Increased pulse
- Anorexia
- Nausea
- Vomiting
- Diarrhea
- Muscle tightness
- Fatigue
- Increased respiratory rate and shortness of breath
- Pallor
- Increased perspiration
- Increased systolic blood pressure
- Pupil dilation
- Dry mouth

Related Factors

Natural/innate origin (e.g., sudden noise, height, pain, loss of physical support)

Learned response (e.g., conditioning, modeling from or identification with others)

Separation from support system in potentially stressful situation (e.g., hospitalization, hospital procedures)

Unfamiliarity with environmental experience(s)

Language barrier

Sensory impairment

Innate releasers (neurotransmitters)

Phobic stimulus

READINESS FOR ENHANCED FLUID BALANCE
(2002, LOE 2.1)

Definition *A pattern of equilibrium between fluid volume and chemical composition of body fluids that is sufficient for meeting physical needs and can be strengthened*

Defining Characteristics

- Expresses willingness to enhance fluid balance
- Stable weight
- Moist mucous membranes
- Food and fluid intake adequate for daily needs
- Straw-colored urine with specific gravity within normal limits
- Good tissue turgor
- No excessive thirst
- Urine output appropriate for intake
- No evidence of edema or dehydration

References

Dabinett, J.A., Reid, K., & James, N. (2001). Educational strategies used in increasing fluid intake and enhancing hydration status in field hockey players preparing for competition in a hot and humid environment: A case study. *International Journal of Sport Nutrition and Exercise Metabolism, 11*(3), 334–348.

Holben, D.H., Hassell, J.T., Williams, J.L., & Helle, B. (1999). Fluid intake compared with established standards and symptoms of dehydration among elderly residents of a long-term-care facility. *Journal of the American Dietetic Association, 99*(11), 1447–1450.

Kleiner, S.M. (1999). Water: An essential but overlooked nutrient. *Journal of the American Dietetic Association, 99*(2), 200–206.

DEFICIENT FLUID VOLUME
(1978, 1996)

Definition *Decreased intravascular, interstitial, and/or intra-cellular fluid. This refers to dehydration, water loss alone without change in sodium.*

Defining Characteristics

- Weakness
- Thirst
- Decreased skin/tongue turgor
- Dry skin/mucous membranes
- Increased pulse rate, decreased blood pressure, decreased pulse volume/pressure
- Decreased venous filling
- Change in mental state
- Decreased urine output
- Increased urine concentration
- Increased body temperature
- Elevated hematocrit
- Sudden weight loss (except in third spacing)

Related Factors

Active fluid volume loss
Failure of regulatory
    mechanisms

EXCESS FLUID VOLUME
(1982, 1996)

Definition *Increased isotonic fluid retention*

Defining Characteristics

- Weight gain over short period of time
- Intake exceeds output
- Blood pressure changes, pulmonary artery pressure changes, increased central venous pressure
- Edema, may progress to anascara
- Jugular vein distention
- Changes in respiratory pattern, dyspnea or shortness of breath, orthopnea, abnormal breath sounds (rales or crackles), pulmonary congestion, pleural effusion

- Decreased hemoglobin and hematocrit, altered electrolytes, specific gravity changes
- S3 heart sound
- Positive hepatojugular reflex
- Oliguria, azotemia
- Change in mental status, restlessness, anxiety

Related Factors

Compromised regulatory
    mechanism
Excess fluid intake
Excess sodium intake

RISK FOR DEFICIENT FLUID VOLUME
(1978)

Definition   *At risk for experiencing vascular, cellular, or intracellular dehydration*

Risk Factors

Factors influencing fluid needs (e.g., hypermetabolic state)

Medication (e.g., diuretics)

Loss of fluid through abnormal routes (e.g., indwelling tubes)

Knowledge deficiency related to fluid volume

Extremes of age

Deviations affecting access, intake, or absorption of fluids (e.g., physical immobility)

Extremes of weight

Excessive losses through normal routes (e.g., diarrhea)

RISK FOR IMBALANCED FLUID VOLUME
(1998)

Definition   *At risk for a decrease, increase, or rapid shift from one to the other of intravascular, interstitial, and/or intracellular fluid. This refers to body fluid loss, gain, or both.*

F

Risk Factors

Scheduled for major
invasive procedures
Other risk factors to be
determined

IMPAIRED Gas EXCHANGE
(1980, 1996, 1998)

Definition *Excess or deficit in oxygenation and/or carbon dioxide elimination at the alveolar-capillary membrane*

Defining Characteristics

- Visual disturbances
- Decreased carbon dioxide
- Tachycardia
- Hypercapnia
- Restlessness
- Somnolence
- Irritability
- Hypoxia
- Confusion
- Dyspnea
- Abnormal arterial blood gases
- Cyanosis (in neonates only)
- Abnormal skin color (pale, dusky)
- Hypoxemia
- Hypercarbia
- Headache upon awakening
- Abnormal rate, rhythm, depth of breathing
- Diaphoresis
- Abnormal arterial pH
- Nasal flaring

Related Factors

Ventilation perfusion imbalance
Alveolar-capillary membrane changes

ANTICIPATORY GRIEVING
(1980, 1996)

Definition *Intellectual and emotional responses and behaviors by which individuals, families, communities work through the process of modifying self-concept based on the perception of potential loss*

Defining Characteristics

- Potential loss of significant object (e.g., people, possessions, job, status, home, ideals, parts and processes of the body)
- Expression of distress at potential loss
- Sorrow
- Guilt
- Denial of potential loss
- Anger
- Altered communication patterns
- Denial of the significance of the loss
- Bargaining
- Alteration in eating habits, sleep patterns, dream patterns, activity level, libido
- Difficulty taking on new or different roles
- Resolution of grief prior to the reality of loss

Related Factors

To be developed

DYSFUNCTIONAL GRIEVING
(1980, 1986, 2004, LOE 2.1)

Definition *Extended, unsuccessful use of intellectual and emotional responses by which individuals, families, and communities attempt to work through the process of modifying self-concept based upon the perception of loss*

Defining Characteristics

- Persistent anxiety
- Depression
- Altered activities of daily living
- Prolonged difficulty coping
- Loss-associated sense of despair

- Intrusive images
- Feelings of inadequacy
- Decreased self-esteem
- Diminished sense of control
- Dependency
- Death anxiety
- Self-criticism

Related Factors

General

Preloss neuroticism
Preloss psychological symptoms
Frequency of major life events
Predisposition for anxiety and feelings of inadequacy
Past psychiatric or mental health treatment

Perinatal

Later gestational age at time of loss

Limited time since perinatal loss and subsequent conception
Length of life of infant
Absence of other living children
Congenital anomaly
Number of past perinatal losses
Marital adjustment problems
Viewing of ultrasound images of the fetus

continued

Dysfunctional Grieving, *continued*

References

Canadian Pediatric Society. (2003). *Guidelines for health care professionals supporting families experiencing a perinatal loss.* Retrieved October 27, 2003, from www.cps.ca/english/statements/FN/fn01-02.htm

Harrigan, R., Naber, M.M., Jensen, K.A., Tse, A. & Perez, D. (1993). Perinatal grief: Response to the loss of an infant. *Neonatal Network—Journal of Neonatal Nursing, 12*(5), 25–31.

Williams, G.B. (2001). Short-term grief after an elective abortion. *Journal of Obstetrics, Gynecology, and Neonatal Nursing, 30,* 174–183.

G

RISK FOR DYSFUNCTIONAL GRIEVING
(2004, LOE 3.1)

Definition *At risk for extended, unsuccessful use of intellectual and emotional responses and behaviors by an individual, family, or community following a death or perception of loss*

Risk Factors

General

Preloss neuroticism

Preloss psychological symptoms

Frequency of major life events

Predisposition for anxiety and feelings of inadequacy

Past psychiatric or mental health treatment

Perinatal

Later gestational age at time of loss

Limited time since perinatal loss and subsequent conception

Length of life of infant

Absence of other living children

Congenital anomaly

Number of past perinatal losses

Marital adjustment problems

Viewing of ultrasound images of the fetus

References

Canadian Pediatric Society. (2003). *Guidelines for health care professionals supporting families experiencing a perinatal loss.* Retrieved October 27, 2003, from www.cps.ca/english/statements/FN/fn01-02.htm

Harrigan, R., Naber, M.M., Jensen, K.A., Tse, A., & Perez, D. (1993). Perinatal grief: Response to the loss of an infant. *Neonatal Network—Journal of Neonatal Nursing, 12*(5), 25–31.

Williams, G.B. (2001). Short-term grief after an elective abortion. *Journal of Obstetrics, Gynecology, and Neonatal Nursing, 30,* 174–183.

DELAYED GROWTH AND DEVELOPMENT
(1986)

Definition   *Deviations from age-group norms*

Defining Characteristics

- Altered physical growth
- Delay or difficulty in performing skills (motor, social, expressive) typical of age group
- Inability to perform self-care or self-control activities appropriate for age

- Flat affect
- Listlessness, decreased response time

Related Factors

Prescribed dependence
Indifference
Separation from significant others
Environmental and stimulation deficiencies

Effects of physical disability
Inadequate caretaking
Inconsistent responsiveness
Multiple caretakers

RISK FOR DISPROPORTIONATE GROWTH
(1998)

Definition *At risk for growth above the 97th percentile or below the 3rd percentile for age, crossing two percentile channels; disproportionate growth*

Risk Factors

Prenatal

Congenital / genetic disorders
Maternal nutrition
Multiple gestation
Teratogen exposure
Substance use / abuse
Maternal infection

Individual

Infection
Prematurity
Malnutrition
Organic and inorganic factors
Caregiver and / or individual maladaptive feeding behaviors
Anorexia
Insatiable appetite
Chronic illness
Substance abuse

Environmental

Deprivation
Teratogen
Lead poisoning
Poverty
Violence
Natural disasters

Caregiver

Abuse
Mental illness, mental retardation, severe learning disability

---

INEFFECTIVE **H**EALTH MAINTENANCE
(1982)

Definition *Inability to identify, manage, and/or seek out help to maintain health*

Defining Characteristics

- Demonstrated lack of knowledge regarding basic health practices
- Demonstrated lack of adaptive behaviors to internal/external environmental changes
- Reported or observed inability to take responsibility for meeting basic health practices in any or all functional pattern areas
- History of lack of health-seeking behavior
- Expressed interest in improving health behaviors
- Reported or observed lack of equipment, financial and/or other resources
- Reported or observed impairment of personal support systems

Related Factors

Ineffective family coping
Perceptual/cognitive impairment (complete/partial lack of gross and/or fine motor skills)
Lack of, or significant alteration in, communication skills (written, verbal, and/or gestural)
Unachieved developmental tasks
Lack of material resources
Dysfunctional grieving
Disabling spiritual distress
Lack of ability to make deliberate and thoughtful judgments
Ineffective individual coping

HEALTH-SEEKING BEHAVIORS (Specify)
(1988)

Definition *Active seeking (by a person in stable health) of ways to alter personal health habits and/or the environment in order to move toward a higher level of health*

Defining Characteristics

- Expressed or observed desire to seek a higher level of wellness
- Demonstrated or observed lack of knowledge about health-promotion behaviors
- Stated or observed unfamiliarity with wellness community resources
- Expression of concern about current environmental conditions on health status
- Expressed or observed desire for increased control of health practice

Related Factors

To be developed

Note. Stable health is defined as achievement of age-appropriate illness-prevention measures; client reports good or excellent health, and signs and symptoms of disease, if present, are controlled.

H

IMPAIRED HOME MAINTENANCE
(1980)

Definition *Inability to independently maintain a safe growth-promoting immediate environment*

Defining Characteristics

Subjective

- Household members express difficulty in maintaining their home in a comfortable fashion
- Household members describe outstanding debts or financial crises
- Household members request assistance with home maintenance

Objective

- Disorderly surroundings
- Unwashed or unavailable cooking equipment, clothes, or linen

- Accumulation of dirt, food wastes, or hygienic wastes
- Offensive odors
- Inappropriate household temperature
- Overtaxed family members (e.g., exhausted, anxious)
- Lack of necessary equipment or aids
- Presence of vermin or rodents
- Repeated hygienic disorders, infestations, or infections

Related Factors

Individual/family member disease or injury
Unfamiliarity with neighborhood resources
Lack of role modeling
Lack of knowledge
Insufficient family organization or planning

Inadequate support systems
Impaired cognitive or emotional functioning
Insufficient finances

Hopelessness
(1986)

Definition   *Subjective state in which an individual sees limited or no alternatives or personal choices available and is unable to mobilize energy on own behalf*

Defining Characteristics

- Passivity, decreased verbalization
- Decreased affect
- Verbal cues (e.g., despondent content, "I can't," sighing)
- Closing eyes
- Decreased appetite
- Decreased response to stimuli
- Increased/decreased sleep
- Lack of initiative
- Lack of involvement in care/passively allowing care
- Shrugging in response to speaker
- Turning away from speaker

Related Factors

Abandonment
Prolonged activity restriction creating isolation
Lost belief in transcendent values/God
Long-term stress
Failing or deteriorating physiological condition

HYPERTHERMIA
(1986)

Definition   *Body temperature elevated above normal range*

Defining Characteristics

- Increase in body temperature above normal range
- Seizures or convulsions
- Flushed skin

- Increased respiratory rate
- Tachycardia
- Warm to touch

Related Factors

Illness or trauma
Increased metabolic rate
Vigorous activity
Medications or anesthesia
Inability or decreased ability to perspire

Exposure to hot environment
Dehydration
Inappropriate clothing

Hypothermia
(1986, 1988)

Definition *Body temperature below normal range*

Defining Characteristics

- Reduction in body temperature below normal range
- Pallor
- Shivering
- Cool skin
- Cyanotic nail beds
- Hypertension
- Piloerection
- Slow capillary refill
- Tachycardia

Related Factors

Exposure to cool or cold environment

Medications causing vasodilation

Malnutrition

Inadequate clothing

Illness or trauma

Evaporation from skin in cool environment

Decreased metabolic rate

Damage to hypothalamus

Consumption of alcohol

Aging

Inability or decreased ability to shiver

Inactivity

H

DISTURBED PERSONAL IDENTITY
(1978)

Definition *Inability to distinguish between self and nonself*

Defining Characteristics
- To be developed

Related Factors
To be developed

FUNCTIONAL URINARY INCONTINENCE
(1986, 1998)

Definition *Inability of usually continent person to reach toilet in time to avoid unintentional loss of urine*

Defining Characteristics

- Amount of time required to reach toilet exceeds length of time between sensing the urge to void and uncontrolled voiding
- Loss of urine before reaching toilet
- May only be incontinent in early morning
- Senses need to void
- Able to completely empty bladder

Related Factors

Psychological factors
Impaired vision
Impaired cognition
Neuromuscular limitations

Altered environmental factors
Weakened supporting pelvic structures

REFLEX URINARY INCONTINENCE
(1986, 1998)

Definition *Involuntary loss of urine at somewhat predictable intervals when a specific bladder volume is reached*

Defining Characteristics

- No sensation of urge to void
- Complete emptying with lesion above pontine micturition center
- Incomplete emptying with lesion above sacral micturition center
- No sensation of bladder fullness
- Sensations associated with full bladder such as sweating, restlessness, and abdominal discomfort

- Inability to voluntarily inhibit or initiate voiding
- No sensation of voiding
- Predictable pattern of voiding
- Sensation of urgency without voluntary inhibition of bladder contraction

Related Factors

Tissue damage from radiation cystitis, inflammatory bladder conditions, or radical pelvic surgery

Neurological impairment above level of sacral or pontine micturition center

STRESS URINARY INCONTINENCE
(1986)

Definition *Loss of less than 50 ml of urine occurring with increased abdominal pressure*

Defining Characteristics
- Reported or observed dribbling with increased abdominal pressure
- Urinary frequency (more often than every 2 hours)
- Urinary urgency

Related Factors
Weak pelvic muscles and structural supports

Degenerative changes in pelvic muscles and structural supports associated with increased age

High intra-abdominal pressure (e.g., obesity, gravid uterus)

Overdistention between voidings

Incompetent bladder outlet

TOTAL URINARY INCONTINENCE
(1986)

Definition *Continuous and unpredictable loss of urine*

Defining Characteristics

- Constant flow of urine at unpredictable times without uninhibited bladder contractions/ spasm or distention
- Nocturia
- Unsuccessful incontinence refractory treatments
- Unawareness of incontinence
- Lack of perineal or bladder filling awareness

Related Factors

Neuropathy preventing transmission of reflex indicating bladder fullness

Trauma or disease affecting spinal cord nerves

Anatomic (fistula)

Independent contraction of detrusor reflex due to surgery

Neurological dysfunction causing triggering of micturition at unpredictable times

URGE URINARY INCONTINENCE
(1986)

Definition   *Involuntary passage of urine occurring soon after a strong sense of urgency to void*

Defining Characteristics

- Urinary urgency
- Bladder contracture/spasm
- Frequency (voiding more often than every 2 hours)
- Voiding in large amounts (>550 cc)
- Voiding in small amounts (<100 cc)
- Nocturia (more than 2 times a night)
- Inability to reach toilet in time

Related Factors

Alcohol

Caffeine

Decreased bladder capacity (e.g., history of PID, abdominal surgeries, indwelling urinary catheter)

Increased fluids

Increased urine concentration

Irritation of bladder stretch receptors causing spasm (e.g., bladder infection)

Overdistention of bladder

RISK FOR URGE URINARY INCONTINENCE
(1998)

Definition *At risk for involuntary loss of urine associated with a sudden, strong sensation or urinary urgency*

Risk Factors

Effects of medications, caffeine, alcohol

Detrusor hyperreflexia from cystitis, urethritis, tumors, renal calculi, central nervous system disorders above pontine micturition center

Detrusor muscle instability with impaired contractility

Involuntary sphincter relaxation

Ineffective toileting habits

Small bladder capacity

DISORGANIZED INFANT BEHAVIOR
(1994, 1998)

Definition *Disintegrated physiological and neurobehavioral responses to the environment*

Defining Characteristics

Regulatory Problems

- Inability to inhibit startle
- Irritability

State-Organization System

- Active-awake (fussy, worried gaze)
- Diffuse/unclear sleep, state-oscillation
- Quiet-awake (staring, gaze aversion)
- Irritable or panicky crying

Attention-Interaction System

- Abnormal response to sensory stimuli (e.g., difficult to soothe, inability to sustain alert status)

Motor System

- Increased, decreased, or limp tone
- Finger splay, fisting or hands to face
- Hyperextension of arms and legs

- Tremors, startles, twitches
- Jittery, jerky, uncoordinated movement
- Altered primitive reflexes

Physiological

- Bradycardia, tachycardia, or arrhythmias
- Pale, cyanotic, mottled, or flushed color
- Time-out signals (e.g., gaze, grasp, hiccough, cough, sneeze, sigh, slack jaw, open mouth, tongue thrust)
- Oximeter reading: Desaturation
- Feeding intolerances (aspiration or emesis)

continued

Disorganized Infant Behavior, *continued*

Related Factors

Prenatal

Congenital or genetic
disorders
Teratogenic exposure

Postnatal

Malnutrition
Oral/motor problems
Pain
Feeding intolerance
Invasive/painful
procedures
Prematurity

Individual

Illness
Immature neurological
system
Gestational age
Postconceptual age

Environmental

Physical environment
inappropriateness
Sensory inappropriateness
Sensory overstimulation
Sensory deprivation

Caregiver

Cue misreading
Cue knowledge deficit
Environmental stimula-
tion contribution

RISK FOR DISORGANIZED INFANT BEHAVIOR
(1994)

Definition   *Risk for alteration in integrating and modulation of the physiological and behavioral systems of functioning (i.e., autonomic, motor, state, organizational, self-regulatory, and attentional-interactional systems)*

Risk Factors

Pain
Invasive/painful
   procedures
Lack of containment/
   boundaries
Oral/motor problems
Prematurity
Environmental
   overstimulation

READINESS FOR ENHANCED ORGANIZED INFANT BEHAVIOR
(1994)

Definition   *A pattern of modulation of the physiologic and behavioral systems of functioning (i.e., autonomic, motor, state-organizational, self-regulatory, and attentional-interactional systems) in an infant that is satisfactory but that can be improved resulting in higher levels of integration in response to environmental stimuli*

Defining Characteristics

- Definite sleep-wake states
- Use of some self-regulatory behaviors
- Response to visual/auditory stimuli
- Stable physiologic measures

Related Factors

Pain
Prematurity

INEFFECTIVE INFANT FEEDING PATTERN
(1992)

Definition   *Impaired ability to suck or coordinate the suck-swallow response*

Defining Characteristics
- Inability to coordinate sucking, swallowing, and breathing
- Inability to initiate or sustain an effective suck

Related Factors
Prolonged NPO
Anatomic abnormality
Neurological impairment/ delay
Oral hypersensitivity
Prematurity

RISK FOR INFECTION
(1986)

Definition *At increased risk for being invaded by pathogenic organisms*

Risk Factors

Invasive procedures

Insufficient knowledge to avoid exposure to pathogens

Trauma

Tissue destruction and increased environmental exposure

Rupture of amniotic membranes

Pharmaceutical agents (e.g., immunosuppressants)

Malnutrition

Increased environmental exposure to pathogens

Immunosuppression

Inadequate acquired immunity

Inadequate secondary defenses (decreased hemoglobin, leukopenia, suppressed inflammatory response)

Inadequate primary defenses (broken skin, traumatized tissue, decrease in ciliary action, stasis of body fluids, change in pH secretions, altered peristalsis)

Chronic disease

RISK FOR INJURY
(1978)

Definition   *At risk of injury as a result of environmental conditions interacting with the individual's adaptive and defensive resources*

Risk Factors

External

Mode of transport or transportation

People or provider (e.g., nosocomial agents; staffing patterns; cognitive, affective, psychomotor factors)

Physical (e.g., design, structure, and arrangement of community, building, and/or equipment)

Nutrients (e.g., vitamins, food types)

Biological (e.g., immunization level of community, microorganism)

Chemical (e.g., pollutants, poisons, drugs, pharmaceutical agents, alcohol, caffeine, nicotine, preservatives, cosmetics, dyes)

Internal

Psychological (affective orientation)

Malnutrition

Abnormal blood profile (e.g., leukocytosis/leukopenia, altered clotting factors, thrombocytopenia, sickle cell, thalassemia, decreased hemoglobin)

Immune-autoimmune dysfunction

Biochemical, regulatory function (e.g., sensory dysfunction)

Integrative dysfunction

Effector dysfunction

Tissue hypoxia

Developmental age (physiological, psychosocial)

Physical (e.g., broken skin, altered mobility)

RISK FOR PERIOPERATIVE-POSITIONING INJURY
(1994)

Definition   *At risk for injury as a result of the environmental conditions found in the perioperative setting*

Risk Factors
Disorientation
Edema
Emaciation
Immobilization
Muscle weakness
Obesity
Sensory/perceptual
  disturbances due to
  anesthesia

DECREASED INTRACRANIAL ADAPTIVE CAPACITY
(1994)

Definition *Intracranial fluid dynamic mechanisms that normally compensate for increases in intracranial volumes are compromised, resulting in repeated disproportionate increases in intracranial pressure (ICP) in response to a variety of noxious and nonnoxious stimuli*

Defining Characteristics

- Repeated increases of >10 mm Hg for more than 5 minutes following any of a variety of external stimuli
- Baseline ICP ≥10 mm Hg
- Disproportionate increase in ICP following single environmental or nursing maneuver stimulus
- Elevated P_2 ICP wave form
- Volume pressure response test variation (volume-pressure ratio 2, pressure-volume index <10)
- Wide amplitude ICP wave form

Related Factors

Decreased cerebral perfusion ≤50–60 mm Hg

Sustained increase in ICP = 10–15 mm Hg

Systemic hypotension with intracranial hypertension

Brain injuries

DEFICIENT KNOWLEDGE (Specify)
(1980)

Definition *Absence or deficiency of cognitive information related to a specific topic*

Defining Characteristics

- Verbalization of the problem
- Inaccurate follow-through of instruction
- Inaccurate performance of test

- Inappropriate or exaggerated behaviors (e.g., hysterical, hostile, agitated, apathetic)

Related Factors

Lack of exposure
Lack of recall
Information misinterpretation

Cognitive limitation
Lack of interest in learning
Unfamiliarity with information resources

READINESS FOR ENHANCED
KNOWLEDGE (Specify)
(2002, LOE 2.1)

Definition *The presence or acquisition of cognitive information related to a specific topic is sufficient for meeting health-related goals and can be strengthened*

Defining Characteristics

- Expresses an interest in learning
- Explains knowledge of the topic
- Behaviors congruent with expressed knowledge
- Describes previous experiences pertaining to the topic

K

References

Crosby, R.A., & Yarber, W.L. (2001). Perceived versus actual knowledge about correct condom use among U.S. Adolescents: Results from a national study. *Journal of Adolescent Health, 28*(5), 415–420.

Meischke, H., Kuniyuki, A., Yasui, Y., Bowen, D.J., Anderson, R., & Urban, N. (2002). Information women receive about heart attacks and how it affects their knowledge, beliefs and intentions to act in a cardiac emergency. *Health Care for Women International, 23,* 149–162.

Taylor, K.L., Turner, R.O., Davis, J.L., Johnson, L., Schwartz, M.D., Kerner, J., & Leak, C. (2001). Improving knowledge of the prostrate cancer screening dilemma among African American men: An academic-community partnership in Washington, DC. *Public Health Reports, 116*(6), 590–598.

SEDENTARY LIFESTYLE
(2004, LOE 2.1)

Definition *Reports a habit of life that is characterized by a low physical activity level*

Defining Characteristics
- Chooses a daily routine lacking physical exercise
- Demonstrates physical deconditioning
- Verbalizes preference for activities low in physical activity

Related Factors

Deficient knowledge of health benefits of physical exercise

Lack of training for accomplishment of physical exercise

Lack of resources (time, money, companionship, facilities)

Lack of motivation

Lack of interest

References

Guirao-Goris, J.A., Moreno, P., & Martínez-Del, P. (2000). Validación del contenido diagnóstico de la etiqueta diagnóstica enfermera "sedentarismo" [Validation of content in the nursing diagnostic label "sedentary"]. *Enferm Clínica, 4*(11), 135–140.

Lizán Tudela, L., & Reig Ferrer, A. (1999). Adaptación transcultural de una medida de la calidad de vida relacionada con la salud: la versión española de las viñetas COOP/WONCA [Transcultural adaptation of a measure relating quality of life to health: The Spanish version of COOP/WONCA]. *Atención Primaria, 23* (2), 75-83.

Vázquez Altuna, J.(1994). Evaluación de la efectividad de un programa de ejercicio físico en la disminución del peso graso [Evaluation of a program of physical exercise in losing weight]. *Atención Primaria, 14*(4), 711–716.

RISK FOR LONELINESS
(1994)

Definition *At risk for experiencing vague dysphoria*

Risk Factors
Affectional deprivation
Social isolation
Cathectic deprivation
Physical isolation

L

IMPAIRED MEMORY
(1994)

Definition *Inability to remember or recall bits of information or behavioral skills.**

Defining Characteristics

- Inability to recall factual information
- Inability to recall recent or past events
- Inability to learn or retain new skills or information
- Inability to determine if a behavior was performed
- Observed or reported experiences of forgetting
- Inability to perform a previously learned skill
- Forgets to perform a behavior at a scheduled time

Related Factors

Fluid and electrolyte imbalance

Neurological disturbances

Excessive environmental disturbances

Anemia

Acute or chronic hypoxia

Decreased cardiac output

*May be attributed to pathophysiological or situational causes that are either temporary or permanent.

IMPAIRED BED MOBILITY
(1998)

Definition *Limitation of independent movement from one bed position to another*

Defining Characteristics

- Impaired ability to
  - Turn side to side
  - Move from supine to sitting or sitting to supine
  - "Scoot" or reposition self in bed
  - Move from supine to prone or prone to supine
  - Move from supine to long sitting or long sitting to supine

IMPAIRED PHYSICAL MOBILITY
(1973, 1998)

Definition *Limitation in independent, purposeful physical movement of the body or of one or more extremities*

Defining Characteristics

- Postural instability during performance of routine activities of daily living
- Limited ability to perform gross motor skills
- Limited ability to perform fine motor skills
- Uncoordinated or jerky movements
- Limited range of motion
- Difficulty turning
- Gait changes (e.g., decreased walking speed, difficulty initiating gait, small steps, shuffles feet, exaggerated lateral postural sway)

- Decreased reaction time
- Movement-induced shortness of breath
- Engages in substitutions for movement (e.g., increased attention to other's activity, controlling behavior, focus on preillness disability/activity)
- Slowed movement
- Movement-induced tremor

Related Factors

Medications
Prescribed movement restrictions
Discomfort, pain
Lack of knowledge regarding value of physical activity
Body mass index above 75th age-appropriate percentile

Sensoriperceptual impairments
Musculoskeletal, neuromuscular impairment
Intolerance to activity/decreased strength and endurance
Depressive mood state or anxiety

Cognitive impairment

Decreased muscle strength, control and/or mass

Reluctance to initiate movement

Sedentary lifestyle, disuse, deconditioning

Selective or generalized malnutrition

Loss of integrity of bone structures

Developmental delay

Joint stiffness or contractures

Limited cardiovascular endurance

Altered cellular metabolism

Lack of physical or social environmental supports

Cultural beliefs regarding age appropriate activity

Note. Suggested Functional Level Classification:

0 = Completely independent

1 = Requires use of equipment or device

2 = Requires help from another person, for assistance, supervision, or teaching

3 = Requires help from another person and equipment or device

4 = Dependent, does not participate in activity

IMPAIRED WHEELCHAIR MOBILITY
(1998)

Definition *Limitation of independent operation of wheelchair within environment*

Defining Characteristics

- Impaired ability to operate manual or power wheelchair on even or uneven surface
- Impaired ability to operate manual or power wheelchair on an incline or decline
- Impaired ability to operate wheelchair on curbs

Note. Specify level of independence.

Nausea
(1998, 2002, LOE 2.1)

Definition   *A subjective unpleasant, wavelike sensation in the back of the throat, epigastrium, or abdomen that may lead to the urge or need to vomit*

Defining Characteristics
- Report of nausea ("sick to my stomach")
- Increased salivation
- Aversion toward food
- Gagging sensation
- Sour taste in mouth
- Increased swallowing

Related Factors

Treatment Related
Gastric irritation:
Pharmaceuticals (e.g., aspirin, nonsteroidal anti-inflammatory drugs, steroids, antibiotics), alcohol, iron, and blood
Gastric distention:
Delayed gastric emptying caused by pharmacological interventions (e.g., narcotics administration, anesthesia agents)
Pharmaceuticals (e.g., analgesics, antiviral for HIV, aspirin, opioids, chemotherapeutic agents)
Toxins (e.g., radiotherapy)

Biophysical
Biochemical disorders (e.g., uremia, diabetic ketoacidosis, pregnancy)
Cardiac pain

continued

Nausea, *continued*

Cancer of stomach or intra-abdominal tumors (e.g., pelvic or colorectal cancers)

Esophageal or pancreatic disease

Gastric distention due to delayed gastric emptying, pyloric intestinal obstruction, genitourinary and biliary distension, upper bowel stasis, external compression of the stomach, liver, spleen, or other organ enlargement that slows the stomach functioning (squashed stomach syndrome), excess food intake

Gastric irritation due to pharyngeal and/or peritoneal inflammation

Liver or splenetic capsule stretch

Local tumors (e.g., acoustic neuroma, primary or secondary brain tumors, bone metastases at base of skull)

Motion sickness, Menière's disease, or labyrinthitis

Physical factors (e.g., increased intracranial pressure, meningitis)

Toxins (e.g., tumor-produced peptides, abnormal metabolites due to cancer)

Situational

Psychological factors (e.g., pain, fear, anxiety, noxious odors, taste, unpleasant visual stimulation)

References

Hogan, C.M., & Grant, M. (1997). Physiologic mechanisms of nausea and vomiting. *Oncology Nursing Forum, 24*(7), 8–12.

Tang, J.H.C. (1998). *Management of chemotherapy induced nausea: Relaxation therapy.* Unpublished research report, The University of Iowa City, Iowa.

Taylor, J.P. (1994). Validation of *altered comfort*: Nausea as experienced by patients receiving chemotherapy. In R.M. Carroll-Johnson & M. Paquette (Eds.), *Classification of Nursing Diagnoses: Proceedings of the Tenth Conference* (pp. 206–207). Philadelphia: Lippincott.

UNILATERAL NEGLECT
(1986)

Definition *Lack of awareness and attention to one side of the body*

Defining Characteristics

- Consistent inattention to stimuli on an affected side
- Does not look toward affected side
- Leaves food on plate on the affected side
- Inadequate self-care
- Inadequate positioning and/or safety precautions in regard to the affected side

Related Factors

Effects of disturbed perceptual abilities (e.g., hemianopsia)
Neurologic illness or trauma
One-sided blindness

N

NONCOMPLIANCE
(1973, 1996, 1998)

Definition *Behavior of person and/or caregiver that fails to coincide with a health-promoting or therapeutic plan agreed on by the person (and/or family and/or community) and healthcare professional. In the presence of an agreed-on, health-promoting or therapeutic plan, person's or caregiver's behavior is fully or partially nonadherent and may lead to clinically ineffective or partially ineffective outcomes.*

Defining Characteristics

- Behavior indicative of failure to adhere (by direct observation or by statements of patient or significant others)
- Evidence of development of complications
- Evidence of exacerbation of symptoms
- Failure to keep appointments
- Failure to progress
- Objective tests (e.g., physiological measures, detection of physiologic markers)

Related Factors

Healthcare Plan

Duration
Significant others
Cost
Intensity
Complexity

Individual Factors

Personal and developmental abilities
Health beliefs, cultural influences, spiritual values
Individual's value system

Knowledge and skill relevant to the regimen behavior
Motivational forces

Health System

Satisfaction with care
Credibility of provider
Access and convenience of care
Financial flexibility of plan
Client-provider relationships

Provider reimbursement of teaching and follow-up

Provider continuity and regular follow-up

Individual health coverage

Communication and teaching skills of the provider

Network

Involvement of members in health plan

Social value regarding plan

Perceived beliefs of significant others

N

IMBALANCED **N**UTRITION: LESS THAN BODY REQUIREMENTS
(1975, 2000)

Definition *Intake of nutrients insufficient to meet metabolic needs*

Defining Characteristics

- Body weight 20% or more under ideal
- Reported food intake less than RDA (recommended daily allowance)
- Pale conjunctival and mucous membranes
- Weakness of muscles required for swallowing or mastication
- Sore, inflamed buccal cavity
- Satiety immediately after ingesting food
- Reported or evidence of lack of food
- Reported altered taste sensation
- Perceived inability to ingest food
- Misconceptions
- Loss of weight with adequate food intake
- Aversion to eating
- Abdominal cramping
- Poor muscle tone
- Abdominal pain with or without pathology
- Lack of interest in food
- Capillary fragility
- Diarrhea and/or steatorrhea
- Excessive loss of hair
- Hyperactive bowel sounds
- Lack of information, misinformation

Related Factors

Inability to ingest or digest food or absorb nutrients due to biological, psychological, or economic factors

IMBALANCED NUTRITION: MORE THAN BODY REQUIREMENTS
(1975, 2000)

Definition *Intake of nutrients that exceeds metabolic needs*

Defining Characteristics

- Triceps skin fold >25 mm in women, >15 mm in men
- Weight 20% over ideal for height and frame
- Eating in response to external cues (e.g., time of day, social situation)
- Eating in response to internal cues other than hunger (e.g., anxiety)
- Reported or observed dysfunctional eating pattern (e.g., pairing food with other activities)
- Sedentary activity level
- Concentrating food intake at the end of the day

Related Factors

Excessive intake in relation to metabolic need

READINESS FOR ENHANCED NUTRITION
(2002, LOE 2.1)

Definition *A pattern of nutrient intake that is sufficient for meeting metabolic needs and can be strengthened*

Defining Characteristics

- Expresses willingness to enhance nutrition
- Eats regularly
- Consumes adequate food and fluid
- Expresses knowledge of healthy food and fluid choices
- Follows an appropriate standard for intake (e.g., the food pyramid or America Diabetic Association guidelines)
- Safe preparation and storage for food and fluids
- Attitude toward eating and drinking is congruent with health goals

N

References

Long, V.A., Martin, T., & Janson-Sand, C. (2002). The great beginnings program: Impact of a nutrition curriculum on nutrition knowledge, diet quality, and birth outcomes in pregnant and parenting teens. *Journal of the American Dietetic Association, 102*(3 Suppl. 1), S86–89.

Murphy, P.W., Davis, T.C., Mayeaux, E.J., Sentell, T., Arnold, C., & Rebouche, C. (1996). Teaching nutrition education in adult learning centers: Linking literacy, health care, and the community. *Journal of Community Health Nursing 13*(3), 149–158.

Satia, J.A., Kristal, A.R., Curry, S., & Trudeau, E. (2001). Motivations for healthful dietary change. *Public Health Nutrition, 4*(5), 953–959.

RISK FOR IMBALANCED NUTRITION: MORE THAN BODY REQUIREMENTS
(1980, 2000)

Definition *At risk for an intake of nutrients that exceeds metabolic needs*

Risk Factors

Reported use of solid food as major food source before 5 months of age

Concentrating food intake at end of day

Reported or observed obesity in one or both parents

Reported or observed higher baseline weight at beginning of each pregnancy

Rapid transition across growth percentiles in infants or children

Pairing food with other activities

Observed use of food as reward or comfort measure

Eating in response to internal cues other than hunger (e.g., anxiety)

Eating in response to external cues (e.g., time of day, social situation)

Dysfunctional eating patterns

IMPAIRED ORAL MUCOUS MEMBRANE
(1982, 1998)

Definition *Disruption of the lips and soft tissue of the oral cavity*

Defining Characteristics

- Purulent drainage or exudates
- Gingival recession, pockets deeper than 4 mm
- Enlarged tonsils beyond what is developmentally appropriate
- Smooth atrophic, sensitive tongue
- Geographic tongue
- Mucosal denudation
- Presence of pathogens
- Difficult speech
- Self-report of bad taste
- Gingival or mucosal pallor
- Oral pain/discomfort
- Xerostomia (dry mouth)
- Vesicles, nodules, or papules
- White patches/plaques, spongy patches, or white curdlike exudate
- Oral lesions or ulcers
- Halitosis
- Edema
- Hyperemia
- Desquamation
- Coated tongue
- Stomatitis
- Self-report of difficulty eating or swallowing
- Self-report of diminished or absent taste
- Bleeding
- Macroplasia
- Gingival hyperplasia
- Fissures, cheilitis
- Red or bluish masses (e.g., hemangiomas)

Related Factors

Chemotherapy

Chemical irritants (e.g., alcohol, tobacco, acidic foods, drugs, regular use of inhalers or other noxious agents)

Depression

Immunosuppression

Aging-related loss of connective, adipose, or bone tissue

Barriers to professional care

Cleft lip or palate

Medication side effects

Lack of or decreased salivation

Trauma

Pathological conditions: Oral cavity (radiation to head or neck)

NPO for more than 24 hours

Mouth breathing

Malnutrition or vitamin deficiency

Dehydration

Infection

Ineffective oral hygiene

Mechanical (e.g., ill-fitting dentures, braces, tubes [endotracheal/ nasogastric], surgery in oral cavity)

Decreased platelets

Immunocompromised

Radiation therapy

Barriers to oral self-care

Diminished hormone levels (women)

Stress

Loss of supportive structures

O

P

ACUTE PAIN
(1996)

Definition *Unpleasant sensory and emotional experience arising from actual or potential tissue damage or described in terms of such damage (International Association for the Study of Pain); sudden or slow onset of any intensity from mild to severe with an anticipated or predictable end and a duration of less than 6 months*

Defining Characteristics

- Verbal or coded report
- Observed evidence
- Antalgic positioning to avoid pain
- Protective gestures
- Guarding behavior
- Facial mask
- Sleep disturbance (eyes lack luster, beaten look, fixed or scattered movement, grimace)
- Self-focus
- Narrowed focus (altered time perception, impaired thought processes, reduced interaction with people and environment)
- Distraction behavior (e.g., pacing, seeking out other people and/or activities, repetitive activities)
- Autonomic responses (e.g., diaphoresis; changes in blood pressure, respiration, pulse; pupillary dilation)
- Autonomic change in muscle tone (may span from listless to rigid)
- Expressive behavior (e.g., restlessness, moaning, crying, vigilance, irritability, sighing)
- Changes in appetite and eating

Related Factors
Injury agents (biological, chemical, physical, psychological)

P

CHRONIC PAIN
(1986, 1996)

Definition *Unpleasant sensory and emotional experience arising from actual or potential tissue damage or described in terms of such damage (International Association for the Study of Pain); sudden or slow onset of any intensity from mild to severe, constant or recurring without an anticipated or predictable end and a duration of greater than 6 months*

Defining Characteristics

- Weight changes
- Verbal or coded report or observed evidence of protective behavior, guarding behavior, facial mask, irritability, self-focusing, restlessness, depression
- Atrophy of involved muscle group
- Changes in sleep pattern
- Fatigue
- Fear of reinjury
- Reduced interaction with people
- Altered ability to continue previous activities
- Sympathetic mediated responses (e.g., temperature, cold, changes of body position, hypersensitivity)
- Anorexia

Related Factors

Chronic physical/
psychosocial disability

P

READINESS FOR ENHANCED PARENTING
(2002, LOE 2.1)

Definition *A pattern of providing an environment for children or other dependent person(s) that is sufficient to nurture growth and development and can be strengthened*

Defining Characteristics

- Expresses willingness to enhance parenting
- Children or other dependent person(s) express satisfaction with home environment
- Emotional and tacit support of children or dependent person(s) is evident; bonding or attachment evident
- Physical and emotional needs of children/dependent person(s) are met
- Realistic expectations of children/dependent person(s) exhibited

References

Bell, R.P., & McGrath, J.M. (1996). Implementing a research-based kangaroo care program in the NICU. *Nursing Clinics of North America, 31*(2), 387–403.

Gielen, A.C., McDonald, E.M., & Wilson, M.E. (2002). Effects of improved access to safety counseling, products, and home visits on parents' safety practices: Results of a randomized trial. *Archives of Pediatric Adolescent Medicine, 156*(1), 33–45.

Long, A., McCarney, S., & Smyth, G. (2001). The effectiveness of parenting programmes facilitated by health visitors. *Journal of Advanced Nursing, 34*(5), 611–620.

P

IMPAIRED PARENTING
(1978, 1998)

Definition *Inability of the primary caretaker to create, maintain, or regain an environment that promotes the optimum growth and development of the child*

Defining Characteristics

Infant or Child

- Poor academic performance
- Frequent illness
- Runaway
- Incidence of physical and psychological trauma or abuse
- Frequent accidents
- Lack of attachment
- Failure to thrive
- Behavioral disorders
- Poor social competence
- Lack of separation anxiety
- Poor cognitive development

Parental

- Inappropriate child care arrangements
- Rejection or hostility to child
- Statements of inability to meet child's needs
- Inflexibility in meeting needs of child or situation
- Poor or inappropriate caretaking skills

- Frequently punitive
- Inconsistent care
- Child abuse
- Inadequate child health maintenance
- Unsafe home environment
- Verbalization of inability to control child
- Negative statements about child
- Verbalization of role inadequacy or frustration
- Inappropriate visual, tactile, auditory stimulation
- Abandonment
- Insecure (or lack of) attachment to infant
- Inconsistent behavior management
- Child neglect
- Little cuddling
- Maternal-child interaction deficit
- Poor parent-child interaction

P

continued

Impaired Parenting, *continued*

Related Factors
Social

Lack of access to resources
Social isolation
Lack of resources
Poor home environment
Lack of family
cohesiveness
Inadequate child care
arrangements
Lack of transportation
Unemployment or job
problems
Role strain or overload
Marital conflict, declining
satisfaction
Lack of value of
parenthood
Change in family unit
Low socioeconomic class
Unplanned or unwanted
pregnancy
Presence of stress (e.g.,
financial, legal, recent
crisis, cultural move)
Lack of, or poor, parental
role model
Single parent
Lack of social support
networks
Father of child not
involved
History of being abusive
History of being abused
Financial difficulties

Maladaptive coping
strategies
Poverty
Poor problem-solving
skills
Inability to put child's
needs before own
Low self-esteem
Relocations
Legal difficulties

Knowledge

Lack of knowledge about
child health maintenance
Lack of knowledge about
parenting skills
Unrealistic expectation
for self, infant, partner
Limited cognitive
functioning
Lack of knowledge about
child development
Inability to recognize and
act on infant cues
Low educational level or
attainment
Poor communication skills
Lack of cognitive readi-
ness for parenthood
Preference for physical
punishment

Physiological

Physical illness

Infant or Child

Premature birth

Illness

Prolonged separation from parent

Not desired gender

Attention deficit hyperactivity disorder

Difficult temperament

Separation from parent at birth

Lack of goodness of fit (temperament) with parental expectations

Unplanned or unwanted child

Handicapping condition or developmental delay

Multiple births

Altered perceptual abilities

Psychological

History of substance abuse or dependencies

Disability

Depression

Difficult labor and/or delivery

Young age, especially adolescent

History of mental illness

High number or closely spaced pregnancies

Sleep deprivation or disruption

Lack of, or late, prenatal care

Separation from infant/child

Note. It is important to reaffirm that adjustment to parenting in general is a normal maturational process that elicits nursing behaviors to prevent potential problems and promote health.

RISK FOR IMPAIRED PARENTING
(1978, 1998)

Definition *Risk for inability of the primary caretaker to create, maintain, or regain an environment that promotes the optimum growth and development of the child*

Risk Factors

Social

Marital conflict, declining satisfaction

History of being abused

Poor problem-solving skills

Role strain/overload

Social isolation

Legal difficulties

Lack of access to resources

Lack of value of parenthood

Relocation

Poverty

Poor home environment

Lack of family cohesiveness

Lack of or poor parental role model

Father of child not involved

History of being abusive

Financial difficulties

Low self-esteem

Lack of resources

Unplanned or unwanted pregnancy

Inadequate child care arrangements

Maladaptive coping strategies

Low socioeconomic class

Lack of transportation

Change in family unit

Unemployment or job problems

Single parent

Lack of social support network

Inability to put child's needs before own

Stress

Knowledge

Low educational level or attainment

Unrealistic expectations of child

Lack of knowledge about parenting skills

Poor communication skills

Preference for physical punishment

Inability to recognize and act on infant cues

Low cognitive functioning

Lack of knowledge about child health maintenance

Lack of knowledge about child development

Lack of cognitive readiness for parenthood

Physiological

Physical illness

Infant or Child

Multiple births

Handicapping condition or developmental delay

Illness

Altered perceptual abilities

Lack of goodness of fit (temperament) with parental expectations

Unplanned or unwanted child

Premature birth

Not gender desired

Difficult temperament

Attention deficit hyperactivity disorder

Prolonged separation from parent

Separation from parent at birth

Psychological

Separation from infant/child

High number or closely spaced children

Disability

Sleep deprivation or disruption

Difficult labor and/or delivery

Young age, especially adolescent

Depression

History of mental illness

Lack of, or late, prenatal care

History of substance abuse or dependence

P

Note. It is important to reaffirm that adjustment to parenting in general is a normal maturational process that elicits nursing behaviors to prevent potential problems and promote health.

RISK FOR PERIPHERAL NEUROVASCULAR DYSFUNCTION
(1992)

Definition *At risk for disruption in circulation, sensation, or motion of an extremity*

Risk Factors

Trauma
Vascular obstruction
Orthopedic surgery
Fractures
Burns
Mechanical compression
  (e.g., tourniquet, cane,
  cast, brace, dressing,
  restraint)
Immobilization

P

RISK FOR POISONING
(1980)

Definition *Accentuated risk of accidental exposure to, or ingestion of, drugs or dangerous products in doses sufficient to cause poisoning*

Risk Factors

External

Unprotected contact with heavy metals or chemicals

Medicines stored in unlocked cabinets accessible to children or confused people

Presence of poisonous vegetation

Presence of atmospheric pollutants

Paint, lacquer, etc., in poorly ventilated areas or without effective protection

Flaking, peeling paint or plaster in presence of young children

Chemical contamination of food and water

Availability of illicit drugs potentially contaminated by poisonous additives

Large supplies of drugs in house

Dangerous products placed or stored within reach of children or confused people

Internal

Verbalization that occupational setting is without adequate safeguards

Reduced vision

Lack of safety or drug education

Lack of proper precaution

Insufficient finances

Cognitive or emotional difficulties

P

POST-TRAUMA SYNDROME
(1986, 1998)

Definition *Sustained maladaptive response to a traumatic, overwhelming event*

Defining Characteristics

- Avoidance
- Repression
- Difficulty in concentrating
- Grief
- Intrusive thoughts
- Neurosensory irritability
- Palpitations
- Enuresis (in children)
- Anger and/or rage
- Intrusive dreams
- Nightmares
- Aggression
- Hypervigilant
- Exaggerated startle response
- Hopelessness
- Altered mood states
- Shame
- Panic attacks
- Alienation
- Denial
- Horror
- Substance abuse
- Depression
- Anxiety
- Guilt
- Fear
- Gastric irritability
- Detachment
- Psychogenic amnesia
- Irritability
- Numbing
- Compulsive behavior
- Flashbacks
- Headaches

Related Factors

Events outside the range of usual human experience

Physical and psychosocial abuse

Tragic occurrence involving multiple deaths

Epidemics

Sudden destruction of one's home or community

Being held prisoner of war or criminal victimization (torture)

Wars

Rape

Natural and/or man-made disasters

Serious accidents

Witnessing mutilation, violent death, or other horrors

Serious threat or injury to self or loved ones

Industrial and motor vehicle accidents

Military combat

P

RISK FOR POST-TRAUMA SYNDROME
(1998)

Definition *At risk for sustained maladaptive response to a traumatic, overwhelming event*

Risk Factors

Exaggerated sense of
   responsibility
Perception of event
Survivor's role in the
   event
Occupation (e.g., police,
   fire, rescue, corrections,
   emergency room staff,
   mental health worker)

Displacement from home
Inadequate social support
Nonsupportive
   environment
Diminished ego strength
Duration of the event

P

POWERLESSNESS
(1982)

Definition *Perception that one's own action will not significantly affect an outcome; a perceived lack of control over a current situation or immediate happening*

Defining Characteristics

Low

- Expressions of uncertainty about fluctuating energy levels
- Passivity

Moderate

- Nonparticipation in care or decision making when opportunities are provided
- Resentment, anger, guilt
- Reluctance to express true feelings
- Passivity
- Dependence on others that may result in irritability
- Fearing alienation from caregivers
- Expressions of dissatisfaction and frustration over inability to perform previous tasks / activities

- Expression of doubt regarding role performance
- Does not monitor progress
- Does not defend self-care practices when challenged
- Inability to seek information regarding care

Severe

- Verbal expressions of having no control
  - Over self-care
  - Or influence over situation
  - Or influence over outcome
- Apathy
- Depression over physical deterioration that occurs despite patient compliance with regimens

Related Factors

Healthcare environment
Illness-related regimen
Interpersonal interaction
Lifestyle of helplessness

P

RISK FOR POWERLESSNESS
(2000)

Definition *At risk for perceived lack of control over a situation and/or one's ability to significantly affect an outcome*

Risk Factors

Physiological

Chronic or acute illness (hospitalization, intubation, ventilator, suctioning)

Acute injury or progressive debilitating disease process (e.g., spinal cord injury, multiple sclerosis)

Aging (e.g., decreased physical strength, decreased mobility)

Dying

Psychosocial

Lack of knowledge of illness or healthcare system

Lifestyle of dependency with inadequate coping patterns

Absence of integrality (e.g., essence of power)

Decreased self-esteem

Low or unstable body image

P

INEFFECTIVE PROTECTION
(1990)

Definition   *Decrease in the ability to guard self from internal or external threats such as illness or injury*

Defining Characteristics

- Maladaptive stress response
- Neurosensory alteration
- Impaired healing
- Deficient immunity
- Altered clotting
- Dyspnea
- Insomnia
- Weakness
- Restlessness
- Pressure ulcers
- Perspiring
- Itching
- Immobility
- Chilling
- Fatigue
- Disorientation
- Cough
- Anorexia

Related Factors

Abnormal blood profiles (e.g., leukopenia, thrombocytopenia, anemia, coagulation)
Inadequate nutrition
Extremes of age
Drug therapies (e.g., antineoplastic, corticosteroid, immune, anticoagulant, thrombolytic)

Alcohol abuse
Treatments (e.g., surgery, radiation)
Diseases such as cancer and immune disorders

Rape-Trauma Syndrome
(1980, 1998)

Definition   *Sustained maladaptive response to a forced, violent sexual penetration against the victim's will and consent*

Defining Characteristics

- Disorganization
- Change in relationships
- Confusion
- Physical trauma (e.g., bruising, tissue irritation)
- Suicide attempts
- Denial
- Guilt
- Paranoia
- Humiliation
- Embarrassment
- Aggression
- Muscle tension and/or spasms
- Mood swings
- Dependence
- Powerlessness
- Nightmares and sleep disturbances
- Sexual dysfunction
- Revenge
- Phobias
- Loss of self-esteem
- Inability to make decisions
- Dissociative disorders
- Self-blame
- Hyperalertness
- Vulnerability
- Substance abuse
- Depression
- Helplessness
- Anger
- Anxiety
- Agitation
- Shame
- Shock
- Fear

Related Factors

Rape

Note. This syndrome includes the following three subcomponents: Rape-Trauma, Compound Reaction, and Silent Reaction. In this text each appears as a separate diagnosis.

Rape-Trauma Syndrome: Compound Reaction
(1980)

Definition *Forced violent sexual penetration against the victim's will and consent. The trauma syndrome that develops from this attack or attempted attack includes an acute phase of disorganization of the victim's lifestyle and a long-term process of reorganization of lifestyle.*

Defining Characteristics

- Change in lifestyle (e.g., changes in residence, dealing with repetitive nightmares and phobias, seeking family support, seeking social network support in long-term phase)
- Emotional reaction (e.g., anger, embarrassment, fear of physical violence and death, humiliation, revenge, self-blame in acute phase)
- Multiple physical symptoms (e.g., gastrointestinal irritability, genitourinary discomfort, muscle tension, sleep pattern disturbance in acute phase)
- Reactivated symptoms of such previous conditions (i.e., physical illness, psychiatric illness in acute phase)
- Reliance on alcohol/ drugs (acute phase)

Related Factors

To be developed

R

Note. This syndrome includes the following three subcomponents: Rape-Trauma, Compound Reaction, and Silent Reaction. In this text each appears as a separate diagnosis.

Rape-Trauma Syndrome: Silent Reaction
(1980)

Definition *Forced violent sexual penetration against the victim's will and consent. The trauma syndrome that develops from this attack or attempted attack includes an acute phase of disorganization of the victim's lifestyle and a long-term process of reorganization of lifestyle.*

Defining Characteristics

- Increased anxiety during interview (i.e., blocking of associations, long periods of silence, minor stuttering, physical distress)
- Sudden onset of phobic reactions
- No verbalization of the occurrence of rape
- Abrupt changes in relationships with men
- Increase in nightmares
- Pronounced changes in sexual behavior

Related Factors

To be developed

Note. This syndrome includes the following three sub-components: Rape-Trauma, Compound Reaction, and Silent Reaction. In this text each appears as a separate diagnosis.

IMPAIRED RELIGIOSITY*

(2004, LOE 2.1)

Definition *Impaired ability to exercise reliance on beliefs and/or participate in rituals of a particular faith tradition*

Defining Characteristics

- Demonstrates or explains difficulty adhering to prescribed religious beliefs and rituals. For example:
  - Religious ceremonies
  - Dietary regulations
  - Clothing
  - Prayer
  - Worship / religious services
  - Private religious behaviors / reading religious materials / media
  - Holiday observances
  - Meetings with religious leaders
- Expresses emotional distress because of separation from fith community
- Expresses emotional distress regarding religious beliefs and / or religious social network
- Expresses a need to reconnect with previous belief patterns and customs
- Questions religious belief patterns and customs

Related Factors

Physical

Sickness / illness
Pain

Psychological Factors

Ineffective support / coping
Personal disaster / crisis

Lack of security
Anxiety
Fear of death
Ineffective coping with disease
Use of religion to manipulate

R

continued

*The DRC recognizes that the term "religiosity" may be culture specific; the concept, however, is well supported by literature in the U.S.

Impaired Religiosity, *continued*

Sociocultural

Barriers to practicing
religion (cultural and
environmental)
Lack of social integration
Lack of social/cultural
interaction

Spiritual

Spiritual crises
Suffering

*Developmental and
Situational*

End-stage life crises
Life transitions
Aging

References

Burkhart, L., & Solari-Twadell, P.A. (2001). Spirituality and religiousness: Differentiating the diagnosis through a review of the
nursing literature. *Nursing Diagnosis: The International Journal of
Nursing Language and Classification, 12,* 45–54.

Chatters, L.M., Taylor, R.J., & Lincoln, K.D. (2001). Advances in the
measurement of religiosity among older African Americans: Implications for health and mental health researchers. *Journal of
Mental Health and Aging, 7*(1), 181–200.

Whitfield, W. (2002). Research in religion and mental health: Naming of parts—Some reflections. *International Journal of Psychiatric
Nursing Research, 8*(1), 891–896.

R

READINESS FOR ENHANCED RELIGIOSITY*
(2004, LOE 2.1)

Definition *Ability to increase reliance on religious beliefs and/or participate in rituals of a particular faith tradition*

Defining Characteristics

- Expresses desire to strengthen religious belief patterns and customs that had provided comfort/religion in the past
- Request for assistance to increase participation in prescribed religious beliefs through:
  - Religious ceremonies
  - Dietary regulations/rituals
  - Clothing
  - Prayer
  - Worship/religious services
  - Private religious behaviors/reading religious materials/media
  - Holiday observances
- Requests assistance expanding religious options
- Requests meeting with religious leaders/facilitators
- Requests forgiveness, reconciliation
- Requests religious material and/or experiences
- Questions or rejects belief patterns and customs that are harmful

continued

R

*The DRC recognizes that the term "religiosity" may be culture specific; the concept, however, is well supported by literature in the U.S.

Readiness for Enhanced Religiosity, *continued*

References

Burkhart, L., & Solari-Twadell, P.A. (2001). Spirituality and religiousness: Differentiating the diagnosis through a review of the nursing literature. *Nursing Diagnosis: The International Journal of Nursing Language and Classification, 12,* 45–54.

Chatters, L.M., Taylor, R.J., & Lincoln, K.D. (2001). Advances in the measurement of religiosity among older African Americans: Implications for health and mental health researchers. *Journal of Mental Health and Aging, 7*(1), 181–200.

Whitfield, W. (2002). Research in religion and mental health: Naming of parts—Some reflections. *International Journal of Psychiatric Nursing Research, 8*(1), 891–896.

RISK FOR IMPAIRED RELIGIOSITY*
(2004, LOE 2.1)

Definition *At risk for an impaired ability to exercise reliance on religious beliefs and/or participate in rituals of a particular faith tradition*

Related Factors

Physical

Illness/hospitalization
Pain

Psychological

Ineffective support/
   coping/caregiving
Depression
Lack of security

Sociocultural

Lack of social interaction
Cultural barrier to prac-
   ticing religion

Social isolation

Spiritual

Suffering

Environmental

Lack of transportation
Environmental barriers
   to practicing religion

Developmental

Life transitions

References

Burkhart, L., & Solari-Twadell, P.A. (2001). Spirituality and religiousness: Differentiating the diagnosis through a review of the nursing literature. *Nursing Diagnosis: The International Journal of Nursing Language and Classification, 12,* 45–54.

Chatters, L.M., Taylor, R.J., & Lincoln, K.D. (2001). Advances in the measurement of religiosity among older African Americans: Implications for health and mental health researchers. *Journal of Mental Health and Aging, 7*(1), 181–200.

Whitfield, W. (2002). Research in religion and mental health: Naming of parts—Some reflections. *International Journal of Psychiatric Nursing Research, 8*(1), 891–896.

R

*The DRC recognizes that the term "religiosity" may be culture specific; the concept, however, is well supported by literature in the U.S.

Relocation Stress Syndrome
(1992, 2000)

Definition *Physiological and/or psychosocial disturbance following transfer from one environment to another*

Defining Characteristics

- Temporary or permanent move
- Voluntary/involuntary move
- Aloneness, alienation, loneliness
- Depression
- Anxiety (e.g., separation)
- Sleep disturbance
- Withdrawal
- Anger
- Loss of identity, self-worth, or self-esteem
- Increased verbalization of needs, unwillingness to move, or concern over relocation
- Increased physical symptoms/illness (e.g., gastrointestinal disturbance, weight change)
- Dependency
- Insecurity
- Pessimism
- Frustration
- Worry
- Fear

Related Factors

Unpredictability of experience
Isolation from family/friends
Past, concurrent, and recent losses
Feelings of powerlessness
Lack of adequate support system/group
Lack of predeparture counseling
Passive coping
Impaired psychosocial health
Language barrier
Decreased health status

RISK FOR RELOCATION STRESS SYNDROME
(2000)

Definition *At risk for physiological and/or psychosocial disturbance following transfer from one environment to another*

Risk Factors

Moderate to high degree of environmental change (e.g., physical, ethnic, cultural)

Temporary and/or permanent moves

Voluntary/involuntary move

Lack of adequate support system/group

Feelings of powerlessness

Moderate mental competence (e.g., alert enough to experience changes)

Unpredictability of experiences

Decreased psychosocial or physical health status

Lack of predeparture counseling

Passive coping

Past, current, recent losses

INEFFECTIVE ROLE PERFORMANCE
(1978, 1996, 1998)

Definition *Patterns of behavior and self-expression that do not match the environmental context, norms, and expectations*

Defining Characteristics

- Change in self-perception of role
- Role denial
- Inadequate external support for role enactment
- Inadequate adaptation to change or transition
- System conflict
- Change in usual patterns of responsibility
- Discrimination
- Domestic violence
- Harassment
- Uncertainty
- Altered role perceptions
- Role strain
- Inadequate self-management
- Role ambivalence
- Pessimistic attitude
- Inadequate motivation
- Inadequate confidence
- Inadequate role competency and skills
- Inadequate knowledge
- Inappropriate developmental expectations
- Role conflict
- Role confusion
- Powerlessness
- Inadequate coping
- Anxiety or depression
- Role overload
- Change in other's perception of role
- Change in capacity to resume role
- Role dissatisfaction
- Inadequate opportunities for role enactment

Related Factors
Social

Inadequate or inappropriate linkage with the healthcare system
Job schedule demands
Young age, developmental level

Lack of rewards
Poverty
Family conflict
Inadequate support system

Inadequate role socialization (e.g., role model, expectations, responsibilities)
Low socioeconomic status
Stress and conflict
Domestic violence
Lack of resources

Knowledge

Inadequate role preparation (e.g., role transition, skill rehearsal, validation)
Lack of knowledge about role, role skills
Role transition
Lack of opportunity for role rehearsal
Developmental transitions
Unrealistic role expectations
Education attainment level
Lack of or inadequate role model

Physiological

Inadequate/inappropriate linkage with health-care system
Substance abuse
Mental illness
Body image alteration
Physical illness
Cognitive deficits
Health alterations (e.g., physical health, body image, self-esteem, mental health, psychosocial health, cognition, learning style, neurological health)
Depression
Low self-esteem
Pain
Fatigue

Note. There is a typology of roles: Sociopersonal (friendship, family, marital, parenting, community), home management, intimacy (sexuality, relationship building), leisure/exercise/recreation, self-management, socialization (developmental transitions), community contributor, and religious.

R

S

BATHING/HYGIENE **S**ELF-CARE DEFICIT
(1980, 1998)

Definition *Impaired ability to perform or complete bathing/hygiene activities for oneself*

Defining Characteristics

- Inability to
  - Wash body or body parts
  - Obtain or get to water source
  - Regulate temperature or flow of bath water
  - Get bath supplies
  - Dry body
  - Get in and out of bathroom

Related Factors

Decreased or lack of motivation
Weakness and tiredness
Severe anxiety
Inability to perceive body part or spatial relationship
Perceptual or cognitive impairment

Pain
Neuromuscular impairment
Musculoskeletal impairment
Environmental barriers

Note. See suggested Functional Level Classification under *Impaired Physical Mobility* (p. 118).

DRESSING/GROOMING Sᴇʟғ-ᴄᴀʀᴇ DEFICIT
(1980, 1998)

Definition *Impaired ability to perform or complete dressing and grooming activities for self*

Defining Characteristics

- Impaired ability to
  - Put on or take off necessary items of clothing
  - Fasten clothing
  - Obtain or replace articles of clothing
- Inability to
  - Put on clothing on upper body
  - Put on clothing on lower body

  - Choose clothing
  - Use assistive devices
  - Use zippers
  - Remove clothes
  - Put on socks
  - Maintain appearance at a satisfactory level
  - Pick up clothing
  - Put on shoes

Related Factors

Decreased or lack of motivation
Pain
Severe anxiety
Perceptual or cognitive impairment
Weakness or tiredness
Neuromuscular impairment
Musculoskeletal impairment
Discomfort
Environmental barriers

Note. See suggested Functional Level Classification under *Impaired Physical Mobility* (p. 119).

S

FEEDING SELF-CARE DEFICIT
(1980, 1998)

Definition *Impaired ability to perform or complete feeding activities*

Defining Characteristics

- Inability to
  - Swallow food
  - Prepare food for ingestion
  - Handle utensils
  - Chew food
  - Use assistive device
  - Get food onto utensil
  - Open containers
  - Ingest food safely
  - Manipulate food in mouth
  - Bring food from a receptacle to the mouth
  - Complete a meal
  - Ingest food in a socially acceptable manner
  - Pick up cup or glass
  - Ingest sufficient food

Related Factors

Weakness or tiredness
Severe anxiety
Neuromuscular impairment
Pain
Perceptual or cognitive impairment

Discomfort
Environmental barriers
Decreased or lack of motivation
Musculoskeletal impairments

Note. See suggested Functional Level Classification under *Impaired Physical Mobility* (p. 119).

S

TOILETING SELF-CARE DEFICIT
(1980, 1998)

Definition *Impaired ability to perform or complete own toileting activities*

Defining Characteristics

- Inability to
  - Get to toilet or commode
  - Sit on or rise from toilet or commode
  - Manipulate clothing for toileting
  - Carry out proper toilet hygiene
  - Flush toilet or commode

Related Factors

Environmental barriers
Weakness or tiredness
Decreased or lack of motivation
Severe anxiety
Impaired mobility status
Impaired transfer ability
Musculoskeletal impairment
Neuromuscular impairment
Pain
Perceptual or cognitive impairment

Note. See suggested Functional Level Classification under *Impaired Physical Mobility* (p. 119).

S

READINESS FOR ENHANCED SELF-CONCEPT
(2002, LoE 2.1)

Definition *A pattern of perceptions or ideas about the self that is sufficient for well-being and can be strengthened*

Defining Characteristics

- Expresses willingness to enhance self-concept
- Expresses satisfaction with thoughts about self, sense of worthiness, role performance, body image, and personal identity
- Actions are congruent with expressed feelings and thoughts
- Expresses confidence in abilities
- Accepts strengths and limitations

References

Carnevale, F.A. (1999). Toward a cultural conception of the self. *Journal of Psychosocial Nursing Mental Health Service, 37*(8), 26–31.

Cole, D.A., Maxwell, S.E., Martin, J.M., Peeke, L.G., Seroczynski, A.D., Tran, J.M., Hoffman, K.B., Ruiz, M.D., Jacquez, F., & Maschman, T. (2001). The development of multiple domains of child and adolescent self-concept: A cohort sequential longitudinal design. *Child Development, 72*(6), 1723–1746.

Walter, R., Davis, K., & Glass, N. (1999). Discovery of self: exploring, interconecting and integrating self (concept) and nursing. *Collegian, 6*(2), 12–15.

S

CHRONIC LOW Self-ESTEEM
(1988, 1996)

Definition   *Long-standing negative self-evaluation/feelings about self or self-capabilities*

Defining Characteristics

- Rationalizes away / rejects positive feedback and exaggerates negative feedback about self (long standing or chronic)
- Self-negating verbalization (long standing or chronic)
- Hesitant to try new things / situations (long standing or chronic)
- Expressions of shame / guilt (long standing or chronic)
- Evaluates self as unable to deal with events (long standing or chronic)
- Lack of eye contact
- Nonassertive / passive
- Frequent lack of success in work or other life events
- Excessively seeks reassurance
- Overly conforming, dependent on others' opinions
- Indecisive

Related Factors

To be developed

S

SITUATIONAL LOW SELF-ESTEEM
(1988, 1996, 2000)

Definition *Development of a negative perception of self-worth in response to a current situation (specify)*

Defining Characteristics

- Verbally reports current situational challenge to self-worth
- Self-negating verbalizations
- Indecisive, nonassertive behavior
- Evaluation of self as unable to deal with situations or events
- Expressions of helplessness and uselessness

Related Factors

Developmental changes (specify)
Disturbed body image
Functional impairment (specify)
Loss (specify)
Social role changes (specify)

Lack of recognition/ rewards
Behavior inconsistent with values
Failures/rejections

S

RISK FOR SITUATIONAL LOW SELF-ESTEEM
(2000)

Definition   *At risk for developing negative perception of self-worth in response to a current situation (specify)*

Risk Factors

Developmental changes
(specify)
Disturbed body image
Functional impairment
(specify)
Loss (specify)
Social role changes
(specify)
History of learned
helplessness
History of abuse, neglect,
or abandonment

Unrealistic self-
expectations
Behavior inconsistent
with values
Lack of recognition/
rewards
Failures/rejections
Decreased power/control
over environment
Physical illness (specify)

S

SELF-MUTILATION
(2000)

Definition *Deliberate self-injurious behavior causing tissue damage with the intent of causing nonfatal injury to attain relief of tension*

Defining Characteristics

- Cuts/scratches on body
- Picking at wounds
- Self-inflicted burns (e.g., eraser, cigarette)
- Ingestion/inhalation of harmful substances/objects
- Biting
- Abrading
- Severing
- Insertion of object(s) into body orifice(s)
- Hitting
- Constricting a body part

Related Factors

Psychotic state (command hallucinations)
Inability to express tension verbally
Childhood sexual abuse
Violence between parental figures
Family divorce
Family alcoholism
Family history of self-destructive behaviors
Adolescence
Peers who self-mutilate
Isolation from peers
Perfectionism
Substance abuse
Eating disorders
Sexual identity crisis
Low or unstable self-esteem

Low or unstable body image
Labile behavior (mood swings)
History of inability to plan solutions or see long-term consequences
Use of manipulation to obtain nurturing relationship with others
Chaotic/disturbed interpersonal relationships
Emotionally disturbed; battered child
Feels threatened with actual or potential loss of significant relationship (e.g., loss of parent/parental relationship)

S

Experiences dissociation or depersonalization

Mounting tension that is intolerable

Impulsivity

Inadequate coping

Irresistible urge to cut/damage self

Needs quick reduction of stress

Childhood illness or surgery

Foster, group, or institutional care

Incarceration

Character disorder

Borderline personality disorder

Developmentally delayed or autistic individual

History of self-injurious behavior

Feelings of depression, rejection, self-hatred, separation anxiety, guilt, depersonalization

Poor parent-adolescent communication

Lack of family confidant

S

RISK FOR SELF-MUTILATION
(1992, 2000)

Definition *At risk for deliberate self-injurious behavior causing tissue damage with the intent of causing nonfatal injury to attain relief of tension*

Risk Factors

Psychotic state (command hallucinations)
Inability to express tension verbally
Childhood sexual abuse
Violence between parental figures
Family divorce
Family alcoholism
Family history of self-destructive behaviors
Adolescence
Peers who self-mutilate
Isolation from peers
Perfectionism
Substance abuse
Eating disorders
Sexual identity crisis
Low or unstable self-esteem
Low or unstable body image
History of inability to plan solutions or see long-term consequences
Use of manipulation to obtain nurturing relationship with others
Chaotic/disturbed interpersonal relationships
Emotionally disturbed and/or battered children
Feels threatened with actual or potential loss of significant relationship
Loss of parent/parental relationships
Experiences dissociation or depersonalization
Experiences mounting tension that is intolerable
Impulsivity
Inadequate coping
Experiences irresistible urge to cut/damage self
Needs quick reduction of stress
Childhood illness or surgery
Foster, group, or institutional care
Incarceration
Character disorders
Borderline personality disorders

S

Loss of control over
problem-solving
situations
Developmentally delayed
or autistic individuals
History of self-injurious
behavior

Feelings of depression,
rejection, self-hatred,
separation anxiety, guilt,
and depersonalization

S

DISTURBED Sensory PERCEPTION (Specify: Visual, Auditory, Kinesthetic, Gustatory, Tactile, Olfactory)
(1978, 1980, 1998)

Definition *Change in the amount or patterning of incoming stimuli accompanied by a diminished, exaggerated, distorted, or impaired response to such stimuli*

Defining Characteristics

- Poor concentration
- Auditory distortions
- Change in usual response to stimuli
- Restlessness
- Reported or measured change in sensory acuity
- Irritability
- Disoriented in time, in place, or with people
- Change in problem-solving abilities
- Change in behavior pattern
- Altered communication patterns
- Hallucinations
- Visual distortions

Related Factors

Altered sensory perception
Excessive environmental stimuli
Psychological stress
Altered sensory reception, transmission, and/or integration
Insufficient environmental stimuli

Biochemical imbalances for sensory distortion (e.g., illusions, hallucinations)
Electrolyte imbalance
Biochemical imbalance

S

SEXUAL DYSFUNCTION
(1980)

Definition   *Change in sexual function that is viewed as unsatisfying, unrewarding, inadequate*

Defining Characteristics

- Change of interest in self and others
- Conflicts involving values
- Inability to achieve desired satisfaction
- Verbalization of problem
- Alteration in relationship with significant other
- Alteration in achieving sexual satisfaction
- Actual or perceived limitations imposed by disease and/or therapy
- Seeking confirmation of desirability
- Alterations in achieving perceived sex role

Related Factors

Misinformation or lack of knowledge
Vulnerability
Values conflict
Psychosocial abuse (e.g., harmful relationships)
Physical abuse
Lack of privacy
Ineffectual or absent role models
Altered body structure or function (e.g., pregnancy, recent childbirth, drugs, surgery, anomalies, disease process, trauma, radiation)
Lack of significant other
Biopsychosocial alteration of sexuality

S

INEFFECTIVE SEXUALITY PATTERN
(1986)

Definition   *Expressions of concern regarding own sexuality*

Defining Characteristics
• Reported difficulties, limitations, or changes in sexual behaviors or activities

Related Factors

Lack of significant other

Conflicts with sexual orientation or variant preferences

Fear of pregnancy or of acquiring a sexually transmitted disease

Impaired relationship with a significant other

Ineffective or absent role models

Knowledge/skill deficit about alternative responses to health-related transitions, altered body function or structure, illness or medical treatment

Lack of privacy

S

IMPAIRED Skin Integrity
(1975, 1998)

Definition *Altered epidermis and/or dermis*

Defining Characteristics

- Invasion of body structures
- Destruction of skin layers (dermis)
- Disruption of skin surface (epidermis)

Related Factors

External

Hyperthermia or hypothermia
Chemical substance
Humidity
Mechanical factors (e.g., shearing forces, pressure, restraint)
Physical immobilization
Radiation
Extremes in age
Moisture
Medications

Internal

Altered metabolic state
Skeletal prominence
Immunological deficit
Developmental factors
Altered sensation
Altered nutritional state (e.g., obesity, emaciation)
Altered pigmentation
Altered circulation
Alterations in turgor (changes in elasticity)
Altered fluid status

S

RISK FOR IMPAIRED Skin INTEGRITY
(1975, 1998)

Definition   *At risk for skin being adversely altered*

Risk Factors

External

Radiation
Physical immobilization
Mechanical factors (e.g., shearing forces, pressure, restraint)
Hypothermia or hyperthermia
Humidity
Chemical substance
Excretions and/or secretions
Moisture
Extremes of age

Internal

Medication
Skeletal prominence
Immunologic factors
Developmental factors
Altered sensation
Altered pigmentation
Altered metabolic state
Altered circulation
Alterations in skin turgor (changes in elasticity)
Alterations in nutritional state (e.g., obesity, emaciation)
Psychogenetic

Note. Risk should be determined by the use of a risk assessment tool (e.g., Braden Scale).

S

SLEEP DEPRIVATION
(1998)

Definition *Prolonged periods of time without sleep (sustained natural, periodic suspension of relative consciousness)*

Defining Characteristics

- Daytime drowsiness
- Decreased ability to function
- Malaise
- Tiredness
- Lethargy
- Restlessness
- Irritability
- Heightened sensitivity to pain
- Listlessness
- Apathy
- Slowed reaction
- Inability to concentrate
- Perceptual disorders (e.g., disturbed body sensation, delusions, feeling afloat)
- Hallucinations
- Acute confusion
- Transient paranoia
- Agitated or combative
- Anxious
- Mild, fleeting nystagmus
- Hand tremors

Related Factors

Prolonged physical discomfort

Prolonged psychological discomfort

Sustained inadequate sleep hygiene

Prolonged use of pharmacologic or dietary antisoporifics

Aging-related sleep stage shifts

Sustained circadian asynchrony

Inadequate daytime activity

Sustained environmental stimulation

Sustained unfamiliar or uncomfortable sleep environment

Non-sleep-inducing parenting practices

Sleep apnea

Periodic limb movement (e.g., restless leg syndrome, nocturnal myoclonus)

Sundowner's syndrome

Narcolepsy

S

continued

Sleep Deprivation, *continued*

Idiopathic central nervous system hypersomnolence
Sleep walking
Sleep terror
Sleep-related enuresis

Nightmares
Familial sleep paralysis
Sleep-related painful erections
Dementia

S

DISTURBED SLEEP PATTERN
(1980, 1998)

Definition *Time-limited disruption of sleep (natural, periodic suspension of consciousness) amount and quality*

Defining Characteristics

- Prolonged awakenings
- Sleep maintenance insomnia
- Self-induced impairment of normal pattern
- Sleep onset >30 minutes
- Early morning insomnia
- Awakening earlier or later than desired
- Verbal complaints of difficulty falling asleep
- Verbal complaints of not feeling well-rested
- Increased proportion of Stage 1 sleep
- Less than age-normed total sleep time
- Dissatisfaction with sleep
- Three or more nighttime awakenings
- Decreased proportion of Stages 3 and 4 sleep (e.g., hyporesponsiveness, excess sleepiness, decreased motivation)
- Decreased proportion of REM sleep (e.g., REM rebound, hyperactivity, emotional lability, agitation and impulsivity, atypical polysomnographic features)
- Decreased ability to function

Related Factors

Psychological

Ruminative presleep thoughts
Daytime activity pattern
Thinking about home
Body temperature
Temperament
Dietary
Childhood onset
Inadequate sleep hygiene
Sustained use of anti-sleep agents
Circadian asynchrony
Frequently changing sleep–wake schedule
Depression
Loneliness
Frequent travel across time zones

S

continued

Disturbed Sleep Pattern, *continued*

Daylight/darkness exposure
Grief
Anticipation
Shift work
Delayed or advanced sleep phase syndrome
Loss of sleep partner, life change
Preoccupation with trying to sleep
Periodic gender-related hormonal shifts
Biochemical agents
Fear
Separation from significant others
Social schedule inconsistent with chronotype
Aging-related sleep shifts
Anxiety
Medications
Fear of insomnia
Maladaptive conditioned wakefulness
Fatigue
Boredom

Environmental

Noise
Lighting
Unfamiliar sleep furnishings
Ambient temperature, humidity
Other-generated awakening
Excessive stimulation
Physical restraint
Lack of sleep privacy/ control
Interruptions for therapeutics, monitoring, lab tests
Sleep partner
Noxious odors

Parental

Mother's sleep-wake pattern
Parent-infant interaction
Mother's emotional support

Physiological

Urinary urgency, incontinence
Fever
Nausea
Stasis of secretions
Shortness of breath
Position
Gastroesophageal reflux

READINESS FOR ENHANCED SLEEP
(2002, LOE 2.1)

Definition *A pattern of natural, periodic suspension of consciousness that provides adequate rest, sustains a desired lifestyle, and can be strengthened*

Defining Characteristics

- Expresses willingness to enhance sleep
- Amount of sleep and REM sleep is congruent with developmental needs
- Expresses a feeling of being rested after sleep
- Follows sleep routines that promote sleep habits
- Occasional or infrequent use of medications to induce sleep

References

Floyd, J.A., Falahee, M.L., & Fhobir, R.H. (2000). Creation and analysis of a computerized database of interventions to facilitate adult sleep. *Nursing Research, 49*(4), 236–241.

Mead-Bennett, E. (1990). Sleep promotion: An important dimension of maternity nursing. *Journal of National Black Nurses Association, 4*(2), 9–17.

Stockert, P.A. (2001). Sleep, health promotion. In P.A. Potter & A.G. Perry (Eds.), *Fundamentals of nursing* (5th ed., pp. 1268–1273). St. Louis, MO: Mosby.

S

IMPAIRED SOCIAL INTERACTION
(1986)

Definition *Insufficient or excessive quantity or ineffective quality of social exchange*

Defining Characteristics

- Verbalized or observed inability to receive or communicate a satisfying sense of belonging, caring, interest, or shared history
- Verbalized or observed discomfort in social situations
- Observed use of unsuccessful social interaction behaviors
- Dysfunctional interaction with peers, family and/or others
- Family report of change of style or pattern of interaction

Related Factors

Knowledge/skill deficit about ways to enhance mutuality
Therapeutic isolation
Sociocultural dissonance
Limited physical mobility

Environmental barriers
Communication barriers
Altered thought processes
Absence of available significant others or peers
Self-concept disturbance

S

SOCIAL ISOLATION
(1982)

Definition   *Aloneness experienced by the individual and perceived as imposed by others and as a negative or threatening state*

Defining Characteristics

Objective

- Absence of supportive significant other(s) (family, friends, group)
- Projects hostility in voice, behavior
- Withdrawn
- Uncommunicative
- Shows behavior unaccepted by dominant cultural group
- Seeks to be alone or exists in a subculture
- Repetitive, meaningless actions
- Preoccupation with own thoughts
- No eye contact
- Inappropriate or immature activities for developmental age/stage
- Evidence of physical/mental handicap or altered state of wellness
- Sad, dull affect

Subjective

- Expresses feelings of aloneness imposed by others
- Expresses feelings of rejection
- Inappropriate or immature interests for developmental age/stage
- Inadequate or absent significant purpose in life
- Inability to meet expectations of others
- Expresses values acceptable to the subculture but unacceptable to the dominant cultural group
- Expresses interests inappropriate to the developmental age/stage
- Experiences feelings of differences from others
- Insecurity in public

continued

S

Social Isolation, *continued*

Related Factors

Alterations in mental status

Inability to engage in satisfying personal relationships

Unaccepted social values

Unaccepted social behavior

Inadequate personal resources

Immature interests

Factors contributing to the absence of satisfying personal relationships (e.g., delay in accomplishing developmental tasks)

Alterations in physical appearance

Altered state of wellness

S

CHRONIC SORROW
(1998)

Definition   *Cyclical, recurring, and potentially progressive pattern of pervasive sadness experienced (by a parent, caregiver, individual with chronic illness or disability) in response to continual loss, throughout the trajectory of an illness or disability*

Defining Characteristics

- Expresses periodic, recurrent feelings of sadness
- Feelings that vary in intensity, are periodic, may progress and intensify over time, and may interfere with the client's ability to reach his/her highest level of personal and social well-being
- Expresses one or more of the following feelings: anger, being misunderstood, confusion, depression, disappointment, emptiness, fear, frustration, guilt/self-blame, helplessness, hopelessness, loneliness, low self-esteem, recurring loss, overwhelmed

Related Factors

Death of a loved one
Experiences chronic physical or mental illness or disability (e.g., mental retardation, multiple sclerosis, prematurity, spina bifida or other birth defects, chronic mental illness, infertility, cancer, Parkinson's disease)

Experiences one or more trigger events (e.g., crises in management of the illness, crises related to developmental stages, missed opportunities or milestones that bring comparisons with developmental, social, or personal norms)
Unending caregiving as a constant reminder of loss

S

SPIRITUAL DISTRESS
(1978, 2002, LOE 2.1)

Definition *Impaired ability to experience and integrate meaning and purpose in life through a person's connectedness with self, others, art, music, literature, nature, or a power greater than oneself*

Defining Characteristics

Connections to Self

- Expresses lack of:
  - Hope
  - Meaning and purpose in life
  - Peace / serenity
  - Acceptance
  - Love
  - Forgiveness of self
  - Courage
- Anger
- Guilt
- Poor coping

Connections With Others

- Refuses interactions with spiritual leaders
- Refuses interactions with friends, family
- Verbalizes being separated from their support system
- Expresses alienation

Connections With Art, Music, Literature, Nature

- Inability to express previous state of creativity (singing / listening to music / writing)
- No interest in nature
- No interest in reading spiritual literature

Connections With Power Greater Than Self

- Inability to pray
- Inability to participate in religious activities
- Expresses being abandoned by or having anger toward God
- Inability to experience the transcendent
- Requests to see a religious leader

S

- Sudden changes in spiritual practices
- Inability to be introspective/inward turning
- Expresses being without hope, suffering

Related Factors

Self-alienation
Loneliness/social alienation
Anxiety
Sociocultural deprivation
Death and dying of self or others

Pain
Life change
Chronic illness of self or others

References

Burkhart, L., & Solari-Twadell, A. (2001). Spirituality and religiousness: Differentiating the diagnoses through a review of the nursing literature. *Nursing Diagnosis: The International Journal of Nursing Language and Classification, 12,* 45–54.

Cavendish, R., Luise, B., Bauer, M., Gallo, M.A., Horne, K., Medefindt, J., & Russo, D. (2001). Recognizing opportunities for spiritual enhancement in young adults. *Nursing Diagnosis: The International Journal of Nursing Language and Classification, 12,* 77–91.

Reed, P. (1992). An emerging paradigm for the investigation of spirituality in nursing. *Research in Nursing and Health, 15,* 349–357.

S

RISK FOR SPIRITUAL DISTRESS
(1998, 2004, LOE 2.1)

Definition *At risk for an impaired ability to experience and integrate meaning and purpose in life through a person's connectedness with self, other persons, art, music, literature, nature, and/or a power greater than oneself*

Risk Factors

Physical
Physical illness
Substance abuse/excessive
 drinking
Chronic illness

Psychosocial
Low self-esteem
Depression
Anxiety
Stress
Poor relationships
Separate from support
 systems
Blocks to experiencing
 love

Inability to forgive
Loss
Racial/cultural conflict
Change in religious rituals
Change in spiritual
 practices

Developmental
Life change
Developmental life
 changes

Environmental
Environmental changes
Natural disasters

References

Burkhart, L., & Solari-Twadell, P.A. (2001). Spirituality and religiousness: Differentiating the diagnoses through a review of the nursing literature. *Nursing Diagnosis: The International Journal of Nursing Language and Classification, 12,* 45–54.

Cavendish, R., Luise, B., Bauer, M., Gallo, M.A., Horne, K., Medefindt, J., & Russo, D. (2001). Recognizing opportunities for spiritual enhancement in young adults. *Nursing Diagnosis: The International Journal of Nursing Language and Classification, 12,* 77–91.

Reed, P.G. (1992). An emerging paradigm for the investigation of spirituality in nursing. *Research in Nursing and Health, 15,* 349–357.

S

READINESS FOR ENHANCED SPIRITUAL WELL-BEING
(1994, 2002, LOE 2.1)

Definition *Ability to experience and integrate meaning and purpose in life through connectedness with self, others, art, music, literature, nature, or a power greater than oneself*

Defining Characteristics

Connections to Self
- Desire for enhanced:
  - Hope
  - Meaning and purpose in life
  - Peace/serenity
  - Acceptance
  - Surrender
  - Love
  - Forgiveness of self
  - Satisfying philosophy of life
  - Joy
  - Courage
- Heightened coping
- Meditation

Connections With Others
- Provides service to others
- Requests interactions with spiritual leaders
- Requests forgiveness of others
- Requests interactions with friends, family

Connections With Art, Music, Literature, Nature
- Displays creative energy (e.g., writing, poetry)
- Sings/listens to music
- Reads spiritual literature
- Spends time outdoors

Connections With Power Greater Than Self
- Prays
- Reports mystical experiences
- Participates in religious activities
- Expresses reverence, awe

continued

S

Readiness for Enhanced Spiritual Well-Being, *continued*

References

Burkhart, L., & Solari-Twadell, A. (2001). Spirituality and religiousness: Differentiating the diagnoses through a review of the nursing literature. *Nursing Diagnosis: The International Journal of Nursing Language and Classification, 12,* 45–54.

Cavendish, R., Luise, B., Bauer, M., Gallo, M.A., Horne, K., Medefindt, J., & Russo, D. (2001). Recognizing opportunities for spiritual enhancement in young adults. *Nursing Diagnosis: The International Journal of Nursing Language and Classification, 12,* 77–91.

Reed, P. (1992). An emerging paradigm for the investigation of spirituality in nursing. *Research in Nursing and Health, 15,* 349–357.

S

RISK FOR SUFFOCATION
(1980)

Definition *Accentuated risk of accidental suffocation (inadequate air available for inhalation)*

Risk Factors

External

Vehicle warming in closed garage

Use of fuel-burning heaters not vented to outside

Smoking in bed

Children playing with plastic bags or inserting small objects into their mouths or noses

Propped bottle placed in an infant's crib

Pillow placed in an infant's crib

Person who eats large mouthfuls of food

Discarded or unused refrigerators or freezers without removed doors

Children left unattended in bathtubs or pools

Household gas leaks

Low-strung clothesline

Pacifier hung around infant's head

Internal

Reduced olfactory sensation

Reduced motor abilities

Cognitive or emotional difficulties

Disease or injury process

Lack of safety education

Lack of safety precautions

S

RISK FOR SUICIDE
(2000)

Definition   *At risk for self-inflicted, life-threatening injury*

Risk Factors

Behavioral.

History of prior suicide
attempt
Impulsiveness
Buying a gun
Stockpiling medicines
Making or changing a will
Giving away possessions
Sudden euphoric recovery
from major depression
Marked changes in
behavior, attitude,
school performance

Verbal

Threats of killing oneself
States desire to die/end
it all

Situational

Living alone
Retired
Relocation,
institutionalization
Economic instability
Loss of autonomy/
independence
Presence of gun in home

Adolescents living in
nontraditional settings
(e.g., juvenile detention
center, prison, half-way
house, group home)

Psychological

Family history of suicide
Alcohol and substance
use/abuse
Psychiatric illness/
disorder (e.g., depres-
sion, schizophrenia,
bipolar disorder)
Abuse in childhood
Guilt
Gay or lesbian youth

Demographic

Age: Elderly, young adult
males, adolescents
Race: Caucasian, Native
American
Gender: Male
Divorced, widowed

S

Physical

Physical illness
Terminal illness
Chronic pain

Social

Loss of important
relationship
Disrupted family life
Grief, bereavement

Poor support systems
Loneliness
Hopelessness
Helplessness
Social isolation
Legal or disciplinary
problem
Cluster suicides

S

DELAYED SURGICAL RECOVERY
(1998)

Definition *Extension of the number of postoperative days required to initiate and perform activities that maintain life, health, and well-being*

Defining Characteristics

- Evidence of interrupted healing of surgical area (e.g., red, indurated, draining, immobilized)
- Loss of appetite with or without nausea
- Difficulty in moving about
- Requires help to complete self-care
- Fatigue
- Report of pain/discomfort
- Postpones resumption of work/employment activities
- Perception that more time is needed to recover

Related Factors

To be developed

S

IMPAIRED SWALLOWING
(1986, 1998)

Definition *Abnormal functioning of the swallowing mechanism associated with deficits in oral, pharyngeal, or esophageal structure or function*

Defining Characteristics

Pharyngeal Phase Impairment

- Altered head positions
- Inadequate laryngeal elevation
- Food refusal
- Unexplained fevers
- Delayed swallow
- Recurrent pulmonary infections
- Gurgly voice quality
- Nasal reflux
- Choking, coughing, or gagging
- Multiple swallows
- Abnormality in pharyngeal phase by swallow study

Esophageal Phase Impairment

- Heartburn or epigastric pain
- Acidic smelling breath
- Unexplained irritability surrounding mealtime
- Vomitus on pillow
- Repetitive swallowing or ruminating
- Regurgitation of gastric contents or wet burps
- Bruxism
- Nighttime coughing or awakening
- Observed evidence of difficulty in swallowing (e.g., stasis of food in oral cavity, coughing/choking)
- Hyperextension of head, arching during or after meals
- Abnormality in esophageal phase by swallow study
- Odynophagia
- Food refusal or volume limiting
- Complaints of "something stuck"
- Hematemesis
- Vomiting

Oral Phase Impairment

- Lack of tongue action to form bolus
- Weak suck resulting in inefficient nippling

continued

S

Impaired Swallowing, *continued*

- Incomplete lip closure
- Food pushed out of mouth
- Slow bolus formation
- Food falls from mouth
- Premature entry of bolus
- Inability to clear oral cavity
- Long meals with little consumption
- Nasal reflux
- Coughing, choking, gagging before a swallow
- Abnormality in oral phase of swallow study
- Piecemeal deglutition
- Lack of chewing
- Pooling in lateral sulci
- Sialorrhea or drooling

Related Factors

Congenital Deficits

Upper airway anomalies
Failure to thrive or protein energy malnutrition
Conditions with significant hypotonia
Respiratory disorders
History of tube feeding
Behavioral feeding problems
Self-injurious behavior
Neuromuscular impairment (e.g., decreased or absent gag reflex, decreased strength or excursion of muscles involved in mastication, perceptual impairment, facial paralysis)
Mechanical obstruction (e.g., edema, tracheostomy tube, tumor)
Congenital heart disease
Cranial nerve involvement

Neurological Problems

Upper airway anomalies
Laryngeal abnormalities
Achalasia
Gastroesophageal reflux disease
Acquired anatomic defects
Cerebral palsy
Internal or external traumas
Tracheal, laryngeal, esophageal defects
Traumatic head injury
Developmental delay
Nasal or nasopharyngeal cavity defects
Oral cavity or oropharynx abnormalities
Premature infants

S

EFFECTIVE THERAPEUTIC REGIMEN MANAGEMENT
(1994)

Definition *Pattern of regulating and integrating into daily living a program for treatment of illness and its sequelae that is satisfactory for meeting specific health goals*

Defining Characteristics

- Appropriate choices of daily activities for meeting the goals of a treatment or prevention program
- Illness symptoms within a normal range of expectation
- Verbalizes desire to manage the treatment of illness and prevention of sequelae
- Verbalizes intent to reduce risk factors for progression of illness and sequelae

Related Factors

To be developed

T

INEFFECTIVE THERAPEUTIC REGIMEN MANAGEMENT
(1992)

Definition *Pattern of regulating and integrating into daily living a program for treatment of illness and the sequelae of illness that is unsatisfactory for meeting specific health goals*

Defining Characteristics

- Choices of daily living ineffective for meeting the goals of a treatment or prevention program
- Verbalizes that did not take action to reduce risk factors for progression of illness and sequelae
- Verbalizes desire to manage the treatment of illness and prevention of sequelae

- Verbalizes difficulty with regulation/integration of one or more prescribed regimens for prevention of complications and the treatment or illness or its effects
- Verbalizes that did not take action to include treatment regimens in daily routines

Related Factors

Perceived barriers
Social support deficit
Powerlessness
Perceived susceptibility
Perceived benefits
Mistrust of regimen and/or healthcare personnel
Knowledge deficit
Family patterns of health care
Family conflict

Excessive demands made on individual or family
Economic difficulties
Decisional conflicts
Complexity of therapeutic regimen
Complexity of healthcare system
Perceived seriousness
Inadequate number and types of cues to action

T

READINESS FOR ENHANCED
THERAPEUTIC REGIMEN MANAGEMENT
(2002, LOE 2.1)

Definition *A pattern of regulating and integrating into daily living a program(s) for treatment of illness and its sequelae that is sufficient for meeting health-related goals and can be strengthened*

Defining Characteristics

- Expresses desire to manage the treatment of illness and prevention of sequelae
- Choices of daily living are appropriate for meeting the goals of treatment or prevention
- Expresses little to no difficulty with regulation/integration of one or more prescribed regimens for treatment of illness or prevention of complications
- Describes reduction of risk factors for progression of illness and sequelae
- No unexpected acceleration of illness symptoms

continued

T

Readiness for Enhanced Therapeutic Regimen
Management, *continued*

References

Bakken, S., Holzemer, W.L., Brown, M., Powell-Cope, G.M., Turner, J.G., Inouye, J., Nokes, K.M., & Corless, I.B. (2000). Relationships between perception of engagement with health care provider and demographic characteristics, health status, and adherence to therapeutic regimen in persons with HIV/AIDS. *AIDS Patient Care and STDs, 14*(4), 189–197.

Dodge, J.A., Janz, N.K., & Clark, N.M. (1994). Self management of the health care regimen: A comparison of nurses' and cardiac patients' perceptions. *Patient Education and Counseling, 23*(2), 73–82.

Schumann, A., Nigg, C.R., Rossi, J.S., Jordan, P.J., Norman, G.J., Garber, C.E., Riebe, D., & Benisovich, S.V. (2002). Construct validity of the stages of change of exercise adoption for different intensities of physical activity in four samples of differing age groups. *American Journal of Health Promotion, 16*(5), 280–287.

T

INEFFECTIVE COMMUNITY THERAPEUTIC REGIMEN MANAGEMENT
(1994)

Definition *Pattern of regulating and integrating into community processes programs for treatment of illness and the sequelae of illness that are unsatisfactory for meeting health-related goals*

Defining Characteristics

- Illness symptoms above the norm expected for the number and type of population
- Unexpected acceleration of illness(es)
- Number of healthcare resources insufficient for the incidence or prevalence of illness(es)
- Deficits in advocates for aggregates
- Deficits in people and programs to be accountable for illness care of aggregates
- Deficits in community activities for secondary and tertiary prevention
- Unavailable healthcare resources for illness care

Related Factors

To be developed

T

INEFFECTIVE FAMILY THERAPEUTIC REGIMEN MANAGEMENT
(1994)

Definition *Pattern of regulating and integrating into family processes a program for treatment of illness and the sequelae of illness that is unsatisfactory for meeting specific health goals*

Defining Characteristics

- Inappropriate family activities for meeting the goals of a treatment or prevention program
- Acceleration of illness symptoms of a family member
- Lack of attention to illness and its sequelae
- Verbalizes difficulty with regulation/integration of one or more effects or prevention of complications
- Verbalizes desire to manage the treatment of illness and prevention of the sequelae
- Verbalizes that family did not take action to reduce risk factors for progression of illness and sequelae

Related Factors

Complexity of healthcare system
Complexity of therapeutic regimen
Decisional conflicts
Economic difficulties
Excessive demands made on individual or family
Family conflict

INEFFECTIVE THERMOREGULATION
(1986)

Definition *Temperature fluctuation between hypothermia and hyperthermia*

Defining Characteristics

- Fluctuations in body temperature above and below the normal range
- Cool skin
- Cyanotic nail beds
- Flushed skin
- Hypertension
- Increased respiratory rate
- Pallor (moderate)
- Piloerection
- Reduction in body temperature below normal range
- Seizures/convulsions
- Shivering (mild)
- Slow capillary refill
- Tachycardia
- Warm to touch

Related Factors

Aging
Fluctuating environmental temperature
Immaturity
Trauma or illness

DISTURBED THOUGHT PROCESSES
(1973, 1996)

Definition *Disruption in cognitive operations and activities*

Defining Characteristics

- Cognitive dissonance
- Memory deficit/problems
- Inaccurate interpretation of environment
- Hypovigilance
- Hypervigilance
- Distractibility
- Egocentricity
- Inappropriate nonreality-based thinking

Related Factors

To be developed

T

IMPAIRED TISSUE INTEGRITY
(1986, 1998)

Definition *Damage to mucous membrane, corneal, integumentary, or subcutaneous tissues*

Defining Characteristics
- Damaged or destroyed tissue (e.g., cornea, mucous membrane, integumentary, subcutaneous)

Related Factors
Mechanical (e.g., pressure, shear, friction)

Radiation (including therapeutic radiation)

Nutritional deficit or excess

Thermal (temperature extremes)

Knowledge deficit

Irritants, chemical (including body excretions, secretions, medications)

Impaired physical mobility

Altered circulation

Fluid deficit or excess

T

INEFFECTIVE TISSUE PERFUSION (Specify Type: Renal, Cerebral, Cardiopulmonary, Gastrointestinal, Peripheral)
(1980, 1998)

Definition *Decrease in oxygen resulting in the failure to nourish the tissues at the capillary level*

Defining Characteristics

Renal

- Altered blood pressure outside of acceptable parameters
- Hematuria
- Oliguria or anuria
- Elevation in BUN/creatinine ratio

Cerebral

- Speech abnormalities
- Changes in pupillary reactions
- Extremity weakness or paralysis
- Altered mental status
- Difficulty in swallowing
- Changes in motor response
- Behavioral changes

Cardiopulmonary

- Altered respiratory rate outside of acceptable parameters
- Use of accessory muscles
- Capillary refill > 3 seconds
- Abnormal arterial blood gases
- Chest pain
- Sense of "impending doom"
- Bronchospasm
- Dyspnea
- Arrhythmias
- Nasal flaring
- Chest retraction

Gastrointestinal

- Hypoactive or absent bowel sounds
- Nausea
- Abdominal distention
- Abdominal pain or tenderness

Peripheral

- Edema
- Positive Homan's sign
- Altered skin characteristics (hair, nails, moisture)
- Weak or absent pulses
- Skin discolorations

- Skin temperature changes
- Altered sensations
- Claudication
- Blood pressure changes in extremities
- Bruits
- Delayed healing
- Diminished arterial pulsations
- Skin color pale on elevations, color does not return on lowering the leg

Related Factors

Hypovolemia
Hypervolemia
Interruption of flow, arterial
Exchange problems
Interruption of flow, venous
Mechanical reduction of venous and/or arterial blood flow
Hypoventilation

Impaired transport of oxygen across alveolar and/or capillary membrane
Mismatch of ventilation with blood flow
Decreased hemoglobin concentration in blood
Enzyme poisoning
Altered affinity of hemoglobin for oxygen

T

IMPAIRED TRANSFER ABILITY
(1998)

Definition   *Limitation of independent movement between two nearby surfaces*

Defining Characteristics

- Impaired ability to transfer
  - From bed to chair and chair to bed
  - On or off a toilet or commode
  - In and out of tub or shower
  - Between uneven levels
  - From chair to car or car to chair
  - From chair to floor or floor to chair
  - From standing to floor or floor to standing

Related Factors

To be developed

Note. Specify level of independence.

T

RISK FOR TRAUMA
(1980)

Definition   *Accentuated risk of accidental tissue injury (e.g., wound, burn, fracture)*

Risk Factors

External

High-crime neighborhood and vulnerable clients

Pot handles facing toward front of stove

Knives stored uncovered

Inappropriate call-for-aid mechanisms for bed-resting client

Inadequately stored combustibles or corrosives (e.g., matches, oily rags, lye)

Highly flammable children's toys or clothing

Obstructed passageways

High beds

Large icicles hanging from the roof

Nonuse or misuse of seat restraints

Overexposure to sun, sun lamps, radiotherapy

Overloaded electrical outlets

Overloaded fuse boxes

Play or work near vehicle pathways (e.g., driveways, lanes, railroad tracks)

Playing with fireworks or gunpowder

Guns or ammunition stored unlocked

Contact with rapidly moving machinery, industrial belts, or pulleys

Litter or liquid spills on floors or stairways

Defective appliances

Bathing in very hot water (e.g., unsupervised bathing of young children)

Bathtub without hand grip or antislip equipment

Children playing with matches, candles, cigarettes, sharp-edged toys

Children playing without gates at top of stairs

Children riding in the front seat in car

Delayed lighting of gas burner or oven

Contact with intense cold

Grease waste collected on stoves

continued

T

Risk for Trauma, *continued*

Driving a mechanically unsafe vehicle

Driving after partaking of alcoholic beverages or drugs

Driving at excessive speeds

Entering unlighted rooms

Experimenting with chemical or gasoline

Exposure to dangerous machinery

Faulty electrical plugs

Frayed wires

Contact with acids or alkalis

Unsturdy or absent stair rails

Use of unsteady ladders or chairs

Use of cracked dishware or glasses

Wearing plastic apron or flowing clothes around open flame

Unscreened fires or heaters

Unsafe window protection in homes with young children

Sliding on coarse bed linen or struggling within bed restraints

Use of thin or worn potholders

Unanchored electric wires

Misuse of necessary headgear for motorized cyclists or young children carried on adult bicycles

Potential igniting of gas leaks

Unsafe road or road-crossing conditions

Slippery floors (e.g., wet or highly waxed)

Smoking in bed or near oxygen

Snow or ice collected on stairs, walkways

Unanchored rugs

Driving without necessary visual aids

Internal

Lack of safety education

Insufficient finances to purchase safety equipment or effect repairs

History of previous trauma

Lack of safety precautions

Poor vision

Reduced temperature and/or tactile sensation

Balancing difficulties

Cognitive or emotional difficulties

Reduced large or small muscle coordination

Weakness

Reduced hand-eye coordination

T

IMPAIRED URINARY ELIMINATION
(1973)

Definition *Disturbance in urine elimination*

Defining Characteristics
- Incontinence
- Urgency
- Nocturia
- Hesitancy
- Frequency
- Dysuria
- Retention

Related Factors
Urinary tract infection
Anatomical obstruction
Multiple causality
Sensory motor impairment

READINESS FOR ENHANCED URINARY ELIMINATION
(2002, LOE 2.1)

Definition *A pattern of urinary functions that is sufficient for meeting eliminatory needs and can be strengthened*

Defining Characteristics

- Expresses willingness to enhance urinary elimination
- Urine is straw colored with no odor
- Specific gravity is within normal limits
- Amount of output is within normal limits for age and other factors
- Positions self for emptying of bladder
- Fluid intake is adequate for daily needs

References

Kilpatrick, J.A. (2001). Urinary elimination, health promotion. In P.A. Potter and A.G. Perry (Eds.), *Fundamentals of nursing* (5th ed., pp. 1408–1411). St. Louis, MO: Mosby.

Palmer, M.H., Czarapata, B.J.R., Wells, T.J., & Newman, D.K. (1997). Urinary outcomes in older adults: Research and clinical perspective. *Urologic Nursing, 17*(1), 2–9.

Pfister, S.M. (1999). Bladder diaries and voiding patterns in older adults. *Journal of Gerontological Nursing, 25*(3), 36–41.

U

URINARY RETENTION
(1986)

Definition *Incomplete emptying of the bladder*

Defining Characteristics
- Bladder distention
- Small, frequent voiding or absence of urine output
- Dribbling
- Dysuria
- Overflow incontinence
- Residual urine
- Sensation of bladder fullness

Related Factors
Blockage
High urethral pressure caused by weak detrusor
Inhibition of reflex arc
Strong sphincter

U

IMPAIRED SPONTANEOUS VENTILATION
(1992)

Definition *Decreased energy reserves result in an individual's inability to maintain breathing adequate to support life*

Defining Characteristics

- Dyspnea
- Increased metabolic rate
- Increased pCO_2
- Increased restlessness
- Increased heart rate
- Decreased tidal volume
- Decreased pO_2
- Decreased cooperation
- Apprehension
- Decreased SaO_2
- Increased use of accessory muscles

Related Factors

Respiratory muscle fatigue
Metabolic factors

V

DYSFUNCTIONAL VENTILATORY WEANING RESPONSE
(1992)

Definition *Inability to adjust to lowered levels of mechanical ventilator support that interrupts and prolongs the weaning process*

Defining Characteristics

Severe

- Deterioration in arterial blood gases from current baseline
- Respiratory rate increases significantly from baseline
- Increase from baseline blood pressure (20 mm Hg)
- Agitation
- Increase from baseline heart rate (20 beats/min)
- Paradoxical abdominal breathing
- Adventitious breath sounds, audible airway secretions
- Cyanosis
- Decreased level of consciousness
- Full respiratory accessory muscle use
- Shallow, gasping breaths
- Profuse diaphoresis
- Discoordinated breathing with the ventilator

Moderate

- Slight increase from baseline blood pressure (<20 mm Hg)
- Baseline increase in respiratory rate (<5 breaths/min)
- Slight increase from baseline heart rate (<20 beats/min)
- Pale, slight cyanosis
- Slight respiratory accessory muscle use
- Inability to respond to coaching
- Inability to cooperate
- Apprehension
- Color changes
- Decreased air entry on auscultation
- Diaphoresis
- Eye widening, wide-eyed look
- Hypervigilance to activities

continued

V

Dysfunctional Vemtilatory Weaning Response, *continued*

Mild

- Warmth
- Restlessness
- Slight increase of respiratory rate from baseline
- Queries about possible machine malfunction

- Expressed feelings of increased need for oxygen
- Fatigue
- Increased concentration on breathing
- Breathing discomfort

Related Factors

Psychological

Patient perceived inefficacy about the ability to wean

Powerlessness

Anxiety: moderate, severe

Knowledge deficit of the weaning process, patient role

Hopelessness

Fear

Decreased motivation

Decreased self-esteem

Insufficient trust in the nurse

Situational

Uncontrolled episodic energy demands or problems

History of multiple unsuccessful weaning attempts

Adverse environment (e.g., noisy, active environment, negative events in the room, low nurse-patient ratio, extended nurse absence from bedside, unfamiliar nursing staff)

History of ventilator dependence >4 days to 1 week

Inappropriate pacing of diminished ventilator support

Inadequate social support

Physiological

Inadequate nutrition

Sleep pattern disturbance

Uncontrolled pain or discomfort

Ineffective airway clearance

V

RISK FOR OTHER-DIRECTED Violence
(1980, 1996)

Definition *At risk for behaviors in which an individual demonstrates that he/she can be physically, emotionally, and/or sexually harmful to others*

Risk Factors

Body language: Rigid posture, clenching of fists and jaw, hyperactivity, pacing, breathlessness, threatening stances

History of violence against others (e.g., hitting someone, kicking someone, spitting at someone, scratching someone, throwing objects at someone, biting someone, attempted rape, rape, sexual molestation, urinating/defecating on a person)

History of threats of violence (e.g., verbal threats against property, verbal threats against person, social threats, cursing, threatening notes/letters, threatening gestures, sexual threats)

History of violent anti-social behavior (e.g., stealing, insistent borrowing, insistent demands for privileges, insistent interruption of meetings, refusal to eat, refusal to take medication, ignoring instructions)

History of violence, indirect (e.g., tearing off clothes, ripping objects off walls, writing on walls, urinating on floor, defecating on floor, stamping feet, temper tantrum, running in corridors, yelling, throwing objects, breaking a window, slamming doors, sexual advances)

continued

Risk for Other-Directed Violence, *continued*

Neurological impairment (e.g., positive EEG, CAT, MRI, neurological findings; head trauma; seizure disorders)

Cognitive impairment (e.g., learning disabilities, attention deficit disorder, decreased intellectual functioning)

History of childhood abuse

History of witnessing family violence

Cruelty to animals

Firesetting

Pre/perinatal complications/abnormalities

History of drug/alcohol abuse

Pathological intoxication

Psychotic symptomatology (e.g., auditory, visual, command hallucinations; paranoid delusions; loose, rambling, or illogical thought processes)

Motor vehicle offenses (e.g., frequent traffic violations, use of a motor vehicle to release anger)

Suicidal behavior

Impulsivity

Availability/possession of weapon(s)

V

RISK FOR SELF-DIRECTED VIOLENCE
(1994)

Definition   *At risk for behaviors in which an individual demonstrates that he/she can be physically, emotionally and/or sexually harmful to self*

Risk Factors

Suicidal ideation (frequent, intense prolonged)

Suicidal plan (clear and specific lethality; method and availability of destructive means)

History of multiple suicide attempts

Behavioral clues (e.g., writing forlorn love notes, directing angry messages at a significant other who has rejected the person, giving away personal items, taking out a large life insurance policy)

Verbal clues (e.g., talking about death, "better off without me," asking questions about lethal dosages of drugs)

Emotional status (hopelessness, despair, increased anxiety, panic, anger, hostility)

Mental health (severe depression, psychosis, severe personality disorder, alcoholism or drug abuse)

Physical health (hypochondriasis, chronic or terminal illness)

Employment (unemployed, recent job loss/failure)

Age 15–19

Age over 45

Marital status (single, widowed, divorced)

Occupation (executive, administrator/owner of business, professional, semiskilled worker)

Conflictual interpersonal relationships

Family background (chaotic or conflictual, history of suicide)

continued

V

Risk for Self-Directed Violence, *continued*

Sexual orientation (bisexual [active], homosexual [inactive])
Personal resources (poor achievement, poor insight, affect unavailable and poorly controlled)

Social resources (poor rapport, socially isolated, unresponsive family)
People who engage in autoerotic sexual acts

V

IMPAIRED WALKING
(1998)

Definition *Limitation of independent movement within the environment on foot*

Defining Characteristics

- Impaired ability to
  - Climb stairs
  - Walk required distances
  - Walk on an incline or decline
  - Walk on uneven surfaces
  - Navigate curbs

Related Factors

To be developed

Note. Suggested Functional Level Classification:
  0 = Completely independent
  1 = Requires use of equipment or device
  2 = Requires help from another person, for assistance, supervision, or teaching
  3 = Requires help from another person and equipment or device
  4 = Dependent, does not participate in activity

WANDERING
(2000)

Definition *Meandering, aimless or repetitive locomotion that exposes the individual to harm; frequently incongruent with boundaries, limits, or obstacles*

Defining Characteristics

- Frequent or continuous movement from place to place, often revisiting the same destinations
- Persistent locomotion in search of "missing" or unattainable people or places
- Haphazard locomotion
- Locomotion into unauthorized or private spaces
- Locomotion resulting in unintended leaving of a premise
- Long periods of locomotion without an apparent destination
- Fretful locomotion or pacing

- Inability to locate significant landmarks in a familiar setting
- Locomotion that cannot be easily dissuaded or redirected
- Following behind or shadowing a caregiver's locomotion
- Trespassing
- Hyperactivity
- Scanning, seeking, or searching behaviors
- Periods of locomotion interspersed with periods of nonlocomotion (e.g., sitting, standing, sleeping)
- Getting lost

Related Factors

Cognitive impairment, specifically memory and recall deficits, disorientation, poor visuoconstructive (or visuospatial) ability, language (primarily expressive) defects

Cortical atrophy
Premorbid behavior (e.g., outgoing, sociable personality; premorbid dementia)
Separation from familiar people and places
Sedation

Emotional state, especially frustration, anxiety, boredom, or depression (agitation)

Over/understimulating social or physical environment

Physiological state or need (e.g., hunger/thirst, pain, urination, constipation)

Time of day

Part 2

TAXONOMY II

2005–2006

Part 2 focuses on the historical development of Taxonomy II; a discussion of the multiaxial structure of Taxonomy II with the three levels of domains, classes, and nursing diagnoses; and the future mapping of the nursing diagnoses in the NANDA, NIC, and NOC (NNN) Taxonomy of Nursing Practice. Figure 2.1 illustrates the schemata of the domains and classes. Table 2.1 shows the placement of the approved nursing diagnoses within Taxonomy II, and Table 2.2 displays the placement of the approved nursing diagnoses within the NNN Taxonomy of Nursing Practice.

History of the Development of Taxonomy II

Following the biennial conference in April 1994, the Taxonomy Committee met to place newly submitted diagnoses into the Taxonomy I revised structure. The committee had considerable difficulty, however, categorizing some of these diagnoses. Given this difficulty and the expanding numbers of submissions at level 1.4 and higher, the committee felt a new taxonomic structure might be viable. This possibility gave rise to considerable discussion as to how this might be accomplished in a scholarly and replicable way.

To begin, the committee agreed to determine if there were categories that arose naturally from the data—i.e., from accepted diagnoses. Round One of a naturalistic Q sort was completed at the 1994 (11th biennial) conference in Nashville, Tennessee. Round Two was completed later and the analysis presented at the 1996 biennial conference in Pittsburgh, Pennsylvania. That Q sort yielded 21 categories, far too many to be useful or practical.

In 1998, the Taxonomy Committee forwarded to the NANDA Board of Directors four Q sorts using different frameworks. Framework #1, reported in 1996, was in the naturalistic style. Framework #2 used Jenny's (1994) ideas. Framework #3 used the Nursing Outcomes Classification (NOC) framework (Johnson & Maas, 1997). Framework #4 used Gordon's (1998) Functional Health Patterns. No one of these was entirely satisfactory, although Gordon's was the best fit. With Gordon's permission, the Taxonomy Committee slightly modified her framework to create Framework Number Five, which was presented to the membership in April 1998 at the 13th biennial conference in St. Louis, Missouri. At that conference, the Taxonomy Committee invited members to sort the diagnoses according to domains that had been selected. By the end of the conference, 40 usable sets of data were available for analysis. During the data collection phase at the conference, members of the Taxonomy Committee took careful notes of the questions asked, the confusion expressed by members, and suggestions made for improvements.

Based on the analysis of the data and the field notes, additional modifications were made to the framework. One domain of the original framework was divided into two to reduce the number of classes and diagnoses falling within it. A separate domain was added for growth and development since the original framework did not contain this domain. Several other domains were renamed better to reflect the content of the diagnoses within them. The final taxonomic structure is much less like Gordon's original, but has reduced misclassification errors and redundancies to near zero. This is a much desired state in a taxonomic structure.

Following the 2002 NANDA, NIC, and NOC conference, the approved nursing diagnoses were placed in Taxonomy II. These included 11 health-promotion nursing diagnoses as well as the revised and newly approved nursing diagnoses. In the future, as new nursing diagnoses are developed and approved, they will be added to the taxonomic structure in the appropriate locations. In January 2003 the Taxonomy Committee met in Chicago and made further refinements to the terminology in Taxonomy II. Following the 2004 NANDA, NIC, and NOC conference in Chicago, the Taxonomy Committee placed the newly approved diagnoses in their appropriate categories.

Structure of Taxonomy II

Scientists, informaticists, and managers of databases are the primary users of actual taxonomic structures. Clinicians are primarily concerned with the diagnoses within the taxonomy and rarely need to use them except for referencing. Familiarity with how the diagnostic language is structured, however, will aid the clinician who needs to find information quickly. Thus, a brief explanation of how the taxonomy is designed will be helpful for an understanding of the diagnoses within it.

Taxonomy II has three levels: domains, classes, and nursing diagnoses. Figure 2.1 depicts the organization of domains and classes in Taxonomy II; Table 2.1 shows Taxonomy II with its 13 domains, 47 classes, and 172 diagnoses. A domain is "a sphere of activity, study or interest" (Roget, 1980, p. 287). A class is "a subdivision of a larger group; a division of persons or things by quality, rank, or grade" (Roget, p. 157). "A nursing diagnosis is a clinical judgment about an individual, family or community response to actual or potential health problems/life processes which provides the basis for definitive therapy toward achievement of outcomes for which a nurse is accountable" (NANDA, 1991, p. 65).

The Taxonomy II code structure is a 32-bit integer (or if the user's data base uses another notation, the code structure is a 5-digit code). This structure provides for the growth and development of the classification structure without having to change codes when new diagnoses, refinements, and revisions are added. New codes are assigned to the nursing diagnoses when they are approved by the Board of Directors upon the recommendation of the Diagnosis Review Committee following an open forum hearing at the biennial conference.

Taxonomy II has a code structure that is compliant with recommendations from the National Library of Medicine (NLM) concerning healthcare terminology codes. The NLM recommends that codes not contain information about the classified concept, as did the Taxonomy I code structure, which included information about the location and level of the diagnosis.

Figure 2.1 Taxonomy II Domains and Classes

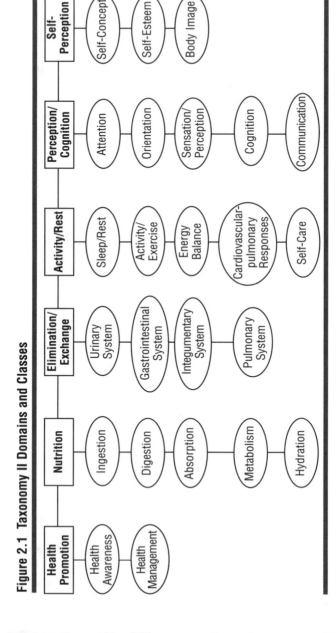

continued

Figure 2.1 *continued*

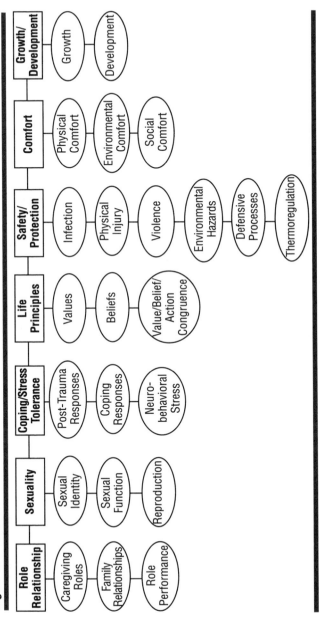

The NANDA taxonomy is a recognized nursing language that meets the criteria established by the Committee for Nursing Practice Information Infrastructure (CNPII) of the American Nurses Association (ANA) (Coenen, McNeill, Bakken, Bickford, & Warren, 2001). The benefit of being included as a recognized nursing language indicates that the classification system is accepted as supporting nursing practice by providing clinically useful terminology. The ANA recognition facilitates the inclusion of NANDA in the ANA Nursing Information and Data Set Evaluation Center (NIDSEC) criteria for clinical information systems (www.nursingworld.org/nidsec/index.htm) and the National Library of Medicine's (NLM) Unified Medical Language System (UMLS; www.nlm.nih.gov/research/umls/unlsmain.html). The taxonomy is registered with Health Level Seven (HL7), a healthcare informatics standard, as a terminology to be used in identifying nursing diagnoses in electronic messages between clinical information systems (www.hl7.org).

NANDA diagnoses have been modeled into SNOMED-CT, which has been accepted as a terminology standard for the U.S. Department of Health and Human Services, the U.S. Consolidated Health Information Initiative, and the United Kingdom's National Health Service. A map of this modeling effort is available from SNOMED International (www.snomed.org).

The Multiaxial System

Taxonomy II was designed to be multiaxial in its form, thereby substantially improving the flexibility of the nomenclature and allowing for easy additions and modifications. An axis, for the purpose of the NANDA taxonomy, is operationally defined as a dimension of the human response that is considered in the diagnostic process.

There are seven axes

Axis 1   The diagnostic concept

Axis 2   Time (acute, chronic, intermittent, continuous)

Axis 3 Subject of the diagnosis (individual, family, group, community)
Axis 4 Age (fetus to old-old adult)
Axis 5 Health status (wellness, risk, actual)
Axis 6 Descriptor (limits or specifies the meaning of the diagnostic concept)
Axis 7 Topology (parts/regions of the body and related functions)

The axes are represented in the named/coded nursing diagnoses through their values. In some cases they are named explicitly, e.g., *ineffective community coping* and *compromised family coping,* in which the subject of the diagnosis (in this instance "community" and "family," Axis 3) is named. "Ineffective" and "compromised" are from the descriptor axis (Axis 6).

In other cases the axis is implicit, e.g., *activity intolerance,* in which the individual (Axis 3) is the subject of the diagnosis. In some instances an axis may not be pertinent to a particular diagnosis, and therefore not a part of the nursing diagnosis label or code. For example, the time axis, which has four values, may not be relevant to each diagnostic situation.

Definitions of the Axes

Axis 1 The Diagnostic Concept

The diagnostic concept is the principal element or the fundamental and essential part—the root—of the diagnostic statement. The diagnostic concept may consist of one or more nouns. When more than one noun is used (e.g., *activity intolerance*), each one contributes a unique meaning as if the two were a single noun; the meaning is different from the nouns stated separately. In some cases an adjective (e.g., spiritual) may be used with a noun (e.g., distress) to denote the diagnostic concept *spiritual distress.*

In other cases, the diagnostic concept and the diagnosis are one and the same. This occurs when the nursing diagnosis is stated at its most clinically useful level and the diagnostic concept adds no meaningful level of abstraction. The diagnostic concepts in Taxonomy II are:

- Activity intolerance
- Adaptive capacity
- Adjustment
- Airway clearance
- Anxiety
- Aspiration
- Attachment
- Autonomic dysreflexia
- Bathing/hygiene self-care
- Bed mobility
- Body image
- Body temperature
- Breastfeeding
- Breathing pattern
- Cardiac output
- Caregiver role strain
- Communication
- Confusion
- Constipation
- Coping
- Death anxiety
- Decisional conflict
- Denial
- Dentition
- Development
- Diarrhea
- Disuse syndrome
- Diversional activity
- Dressing/grooming self-care
- Dysreflexia
- Elimination
- Energy field
- Environmental interpretation
- Failure to thrive
- Falls
- Family processes
- Family processes: Alcoholism
- Fatigue
- Fear
- Feeding self-care
- Fluid balance
- Fluid volume
- Functional incontinence
- Gas exchange
- Grieving
- Growth
- Health maintenance
- Health-seeking behaviors
- Home maintenance
- Hopelessness
- Hyperthermia
- Hypothermia
- Identity
- Incontinence
- Infant behavior
- Infant feeding pattern
- Infection
- Injury
- Intracranial adaptive behavior
- Knowledge
- Latex allergy response
- Less than nutrition requirements
- Loneliness
- Memory
- Mobility

- More than nutrition requirements
- Nausea
- Neurovascular function
- Noncompliance
- Nutrition
- Oral mucous membranes
- Other-directed violence
- Pain
- Parent/infant/child attachment
- Parental role conflict
- Parenting
- Perioperative-positioning injury
- Peripheral neurovascular dysfunction
- Physical mobility
- Poisoning
- Post-trauma
- Powerlessness
- Protection
- Rape-trauma syndrome
- Rape-trauma compound reaction
- Rape-trauma silent reaction
- Reflex incontinence
- Religiosity
- Relocation stress
- Retention
- Role conflict
- Role performance
- Sedentary lifestyle
- Self-care
- Self-care deficit
- Self-concept
- Self-directed violence
- Self-esteem
- Self-mutilation
- Sensory perception
- Sexual dysfunction
- Sexual function
- Sexuality patterns
- Skin integrity
- Sleep
- Sleep deprivation
- Sleep pattern
- Social interaction
- Social isolation
- Sorrow
- Spiritual distress
- Spiritual well-being
- Spontaneous ventilation
- Stress incontinence
- Sudden infant death syndrome
- Suicide
- Suffocation
- Surgical recovery
- Swallowing
- Therapeutic regimen management
- Thermoregulation
- Thought process
- Tissue integrity
- Tissue perfusion
- Toileting self-care
- Total incontinence
- Transfer
- Transfer ability
- Trauma
- Unilateral neglect
- Urge incontinence
- Urinary elimination
- Urinary retention

- Ventilatory weaning response
- Verbal communication
- Violence
- Walking
- Wandering

Axis 2 Time

Time is defined as the duration of a period or interval. The values in Axis 2 are

- *Acute:* Lasting less than 6 months
- *Chronic:* Lasting more than 6 months
- *Intermittent:* Stopping or starting again at intervals, periodic, cyclic
- *Continuous:* Uninterrupted, going on without stop

Axis 3 Subject of the Diagnosis

The subject of diagnosis is defined as the person for whom a diagnosis is determined. Values in Axis 3 are

- *Individual:* A single human being distinct from others, a person.
- *Family:* Two or more people having continuous or sustained relationships, perceiving reciprocal obligations, sensing common meaning, and sharing certain obligations toward others; related by blood and/or choice.
- *Group:* A number of people with shared characteristics.
- *Community:* A group of people living in the same locale under the same governance. Examples include neighborhoods and cities.

When the subject of the diagnosis is not explicitly stated, it becomes the individual by default.

Axis 4 Age

Age is defined as the length of time or interval during which an individual has existed. Values in Axis 4 are

- Fetus
- Neonate
- Infant
- Toddler
- Pre-school child
- School-age child
- Adolescent
- Young adult
- Middle-age adult
- Young old adult
- Middle old adult
- Old-old adult

Axis 5 Health Status

Health status is defined as the position or rank on the health continuum of wellness to illness (or death). Values in Axis 5 are

- *Wellness:* The quality or state of being healthy, especially as a result of deliberate effort.
- *Risk:* Vulnerability, especially as a result of exposure to factors that increase the chance of injury or loss.
- *Actual:* Existing in fact or reality, existing at the present time.

Axis 6 Descriptor

A descriptor or modifier is defined as a judgment that limits or specifies the meaning of a nursing diagnosis. Values in Axis 6 are

- *Ability:* Capacity to do or act
- *Anticipatory:* To realize beforehand, foresee
- *Balance:* In a state of equilibrium
- *Compromised:* To make vulnerable to threat
- *Decreased:* Lessened; lesser in size, amount, or degree
- *Deficient:* Inadequate in amount, quality, or degree; not sufficient; incomplete
- *Defensive:* Used or intended to protect from a perceived threat
- *Delayed:* To postpone, impede, retard

- *Depleted:* Emptied wholly or in part, exhausted of
- *Disproportionate:* Not consistent with a standard
- *Disabling:* To make unable or unfit, to incapacitate
- *Disorganized:* To destroy the systematic arrangement
- *Disturbed:* Agitated or interrupted, interfered with
- *Dysfunctional:* Abnormal, incomplete functioning
- *Effective:* Producing the intended or expected effect
- *Excessive:* Characterized by an amount or quantity that is greater than necessary, desirable, or useful
- *Functional:* Normal complete functioning
- *Imbalanced:* In a state of disequilibrium
- *Impaired:* Made worse, weakened, damaged, reduced, deteriorated
- *Inability:* Incapacity to do or act
- *Increased:* Greater in size, amount, or degree
- *Ineffective:* Not producing the desired effect
- *Interrupted:* To break the continuity or uniformity
- *Low:* Containing less than the norm
- *Organized:* To form as into a systematic arrangement
- *Perceived:* To become aware of by means of the senses; assignment of meaning
- *Readiness for enhanced* (for use with wellness diagnoses): To make greater, to increase in quality, to attain the more desired
- *Situational:* Related to particular circumstance(s)
- *Total:* Complete, to the greatest extent or degree

Axis 7 Topology

The topology consists of parts/regions of the body and/or their related functions—all tissues, organs, anatomical sites or structures. Values in Axis 7 are

- Auditory
- Bladder
- Cardiopulmonary
- Cerebral
- Gastrointestinal
- Gustatory

- Intracranial
- Mucous membranes
- Oral
- Olfactory
- Peripheral neurovascular

- Peripheral vascular
- Renal
- Skin
- Tactile
- Visual

Construction of a Nursing Diagnostic Statement

Because it is a multiaxial framework, the user will notice that the descriptors (e.g., decreased, impaired) now appear on an axis (Axis 6) separate from the diagnostic concepts. As the taxonomy develops, the user may choose the diagnostic concept (Axis 1) that is the clinical judgment about an individual, family, or community; the user may choose the descriptor from those available on the descriptor axis (Axis 6). For example, if the concept of concern is parenting, the user has a choice from the descriptor axis of "impaired" or "readiness for enhanced." In addition, the user has five other axes from which to choose appropriate terms. For the parenting diagnosis, the user might choose "individual" from the unit of care axis (Axis 3), "adolescent" from the age axis (Axis 4) and "risk for" from the health status axis (Axis 5) to arrive at the diagnosis of *risk for impaired individual adolescent parenting.*

Some words of caution as well as encouragement: Using a multiaxial structure allows many diagnoses to be constructed that have no defining characteristics and may even be nonsense (such as "impaired activities of daily living, fetus"). We urge you to use only those diagnoses that are approved for testing and thus have defining characteristics.

The NNN Taxonomy of Nursing Practice

NANDA's Taxonomy II appeared for the first time in *NANDA Nursing Diagnoses: Definitions and Classification, 2001–2002.* The taxonomy is used for the classification of nursing diagnoses. During this period, NANDA began to negotiate an alliance with the Classification Center at the College of Nursing, University of Iowa, Iowa City, Iowa. As a part of that alliance, the possibility of developing a common taxonomic

(text continues on p. 250)

Table 2.1 Taxonomy II: Domains, Classes, and Diagnoses

Domain 1 Health Promotion
The awareness of well-being or normality of function and the strategies used to maintain control of and enhance that well-being or normality of function

Class 1 Health Awareness Recognition of normal function and well-being

Class 2 Health Management Identifying, controlling, performing, and integrating activities to maintain health and well-being

Approved Diagnoses
00082	*Effective therapeutic regimen management*
00078	*Ineffective therapeutic regimen management*
00080	*Ineffective family therapeutic regimen management*
00081	*Ineffective community therapeutic regimen management*
00084	*Health-seeking behaviors (specify)*
00099	*Ineffective health maintenance*
00098	*Impaired home maintenance*
00162	*Readiness for enhanced therapeutic regimen management*
00163	*Readiness for enhanced nutrition*

Domain 2 Nutrition
The activities of taking in, assimilating, and using nutrients for the purposes of tissue maintenance, tissue repair, and the production of energy

Class 1 Ingestion Taking food or nutrients into the body

Approved Diagnoses
00107	*Ineffective infant feeding pattern*
00103	*Impaired swallowing*
00002	*Imbalanced nutrition: Less than body requirements*
00001	*Imbalanced nutrition: More than body requirements*
00003	*Risk for imbalanced nutrition: More than body requirements*

Class 2 Digestion The physical and chemical activities that convert food-stuffs into substances suitable for absorption and assimilation

Class 3 Absorption The act of taking up nutrients through body tissues

Class 4 Metabolism The chemical and physical processes occurring in living organisms and cells for the development and use of protoplasm, production of waste and energy, with the release of energy for all vital processes

Class 5 Hydration The taking in and absorption of fluids and electrolytes

Approved Diagnoses
00027	*Deficient fluid volume*
00028	*Risk for deficient fluid volume*
00026	*Excess fluid volume*
00025	*Risk for imbalanced fluid volume*
00160	*Readiness for enhanced fluid balance*

Domain 3 Elimination and Exchange
Secretion and excretion of waste products from the body

Class 1 Urinary Function The process of secretion, reabsorption, and excretion of urine

Approved Diagnoses
00016	*Impaired urinary elimination*
00023	*Urinary retention*
00021	*Total urinary incontinence*
00020	*Functional urinary incontinence*
00017	*Stress urinary incontinence*
00019	*Urge urinary incontinence*
00018	*Reflex urinary incontinence*
00022	*Risk for urge urinary incontinence*
00166	*Readiness for enhanced urinary elimination*

Class 2 Gastrointestinal Function The process of absorption and excretion of the end products of digestion

Approved Diagnoses
00014	*Bowel incontinence*
00013	*Diarrhea*
00011	*Constipation*
00015	*Risk for constipation*
00012	*Perceived constipation*

continued

Table 2.1 *continued*

Class 3 Integumentary Function The process of secretion and excretion through the skin

Class 4 Respiratory Function The process of exchange of gases and removal of the end products of metabolism

Approved Diagnoses
00030   Impaired gas exchange

Domain 4 Activity/Rest
The production, conservation, expenditure, or balance of energy resources

Class 1 Sleep/Rest Slumber, repose, ease, relaxation, or inactivity

Approved Diagnoses
00095   Disturbed sleep pattern
00096   Sleep deprivation
00165   Readiness for enhanced sleep

Class 2 Activity/Exercise Moving parts of the body (mobility), doing work, or performing actions often (but not always) against resistance

Approved Diagnoses
00040   Risk for disuse syndrome
00085   Impaired physical mobility
00091   Impaired bed mobility
00089   Impaired wheelchair mobility
00090   Impaired transfer ability
00088   Impaired walking
00097   Deficient diversional activity
00100   Delayed surgical recovery
00168   Sedentary lifestyle

Class 3 Energy Balance A dynamic state of harmony between intake and expenditure of resources

Approved Diagnoses
00050   Energy field disturbance
00093   Fatigue

Class 4 Cardiovascular/Pulmonary Responses Cardiopulmonary mechanisms that support activity/rest

Approved Diagnoses

00029	*Decreased cardiac output*
00033	*Impaired spontaneous ventilation*
00032	*Ineffective breathing pattern*
00092	*Activity intolerance*
00094	*Risk for activity intolerance*
00034	*Dysfunctional ventilatory weaning response*
00024	*Ineffective tissue perfusion (specify type: renal, cerebral, cardiopulmonary, gastrointestinal, peripheral)*

Class 5. Self-Care Ability to perform activities to care for one's body and bodily functions

Approved Diagnoses

00109 Dressing/grooming self-care deficit
00108 Bathing/hygiene self-care deficit
00102 Feeding self-care deficit
00110 Toileting self-care deficit

Domain 5 Perception/Cognition

The human information processing system including attention, orientation, sensation, perception, cognition, and communication

Class 1 Attention Mental readiness to notice or observe

Approved Diagnoses
00123   Unilateral neglect

Class 2 Orientation Awareness of time, place, and person

Approved Diagnoses

00127	*Impaired environmental interpretation syndrome*
00154	*Wandering*

Class 3 Sensation/Perception Receiving information through the senses of touch, taste, smell, vision, hearing, and kinesthesia and the comprehension of sense data resulting in naming, associating, and/or pattern recognition

continued

Table 2.1 *continued*

Approved Diagnoses

00122 Disturbed sensory perception (specify: visual, auditory, kinesthetic, gustatory, tactile)

Class 4 Cognition Use of memory, learning, thinking, problem solving, abstraction, judgment, insight, intellectual capacity, calculation, and language

Approved Diagnoses

00126 Deficient knowledge (specify)
00161 Readiness for enhanced knowledge (specify)
00128 Acute confusion
00129 Chronic confusion
00131 Impaired memory
00130 Disturbed thought processes

Class 5 Communication Sending and receiving verbal and nonverbal information

Approved Diagnoses

00051 Impaired verbal communication
00157 Readiness for enhanced communication

Domain 6 Self-Perception
Awareness about the self

Class 1 Self-Concept The perception(s) about the total self

Approved Diagnoses

00121 Disturbed personal identity
00125 Powerlessness
00152 Risk for powerlessness
00124 Hopelessness
00054 Risk for loneliness
00167 Readiness for enhanced self-concept

Class 2 Self-Esteem Assessment of one's own worth, capability, significance, and success

Approved Diagnoses

00119 Chronic low self-esteem
00120 Situational low self-esteem
00153 Risk for situational low self-esteem

Class 3 ***Body Image*** A mental image of one's own body

Approved Diagnoses
00118   Disturbed body image

Domain 7 Role Relationships
The positive and negative connections or associations between people or groups of people and the means by which those connections are demonstrated

Class 1 ***Caregiving Roles*** Socially expected behavior patterns by people providing care who are not healthcare professionals

Approved Diagnoses
00061   Caregiver role strain
00062   Risk for caregiver role strain
00056   Impaired parenting
00057   Risk for impaired parenting
00164   Readiness for enhanced parenting

Class 2 ***Family Relationships*** Associations of people who are biologically related or related by choice

Approved Diagnoses
00060   Interrupted family processes
00159   Readiness for enhanced family processes
00063   Dysfunctional family processes: Alcoholism
00058   Risk for impaired parent/infant/child attachment

Class 3 ***Role Performance*** Quality of functioning in socially expected behavior patterns

Approved Diagnoses
00106   Effective breastfeeding
00104   Ineffective breastfeeding
00105   Interrupted breastfeeding
00055   Ineffective role performance
00064   Parental role conflict
00052   Impaired social interaction

continued

Table 2.1 *continued*

Domain 8 Sexuality
Sexual identity, sexual function, and reproduction

*Class 1 **Sexual Identity*** The state of being a specific person in regard to sexuality and/or gender

*Class 2 **Sexual Function*** The capacity or ability to participate in sexual activities

Approved Diagnoses
00059	*Sexual dysfunction*
00065	*Ineffective sexuality pattern*

*Class 3 **Reproduction*** Any process by which human beings are produced

Domain 9 Coping/Stress Tolerance
Contending with life events/life processes

*Class 1 **Post-Trauma Responses*** Reactions occurring after physical or psychological trauma

Approved Diagnoses
00114	*Relocation stress syndrome*
00149	*Risk for relocation stress syndrome*
00142	*Rape-trauma syndrome*
00144	*Rape-trauma syndrome: Silent reaction*
00143	*Rape-trauma syndrome: Compound reaction*
00141	*Post-trauma syndrome*
00145	*Risk for post-trauma syndrome*

*Class 2 **Coping Responses*** The process of managing environmental stress

Approved Diagnoses
00148	*Fear*
00146	*Anxiety*
00147	*Death anxiety*
00137	*Chronic sorrow*
00072	*Ineffective denial*
00136	*Anticipatory grieving*
00135	*Dysfunctional grieving*
00070	*Impaired adjustment*
00069	*Ineffective coping*

00073	Disabled family coping
00074	Compromised family coping
00071	Defensive coping
00077	Ineffective community coping
00158	Readiness for enhanced coping (individual)
00075	Readiness for enhanced family coping
00076	Readiness for enhanced community coping
00172	Risk for dysfunctional grieving

Class 3 Neurobehavioral Stress Behavioral responses reflecting nerve and brain function

Approved Diagnoses

00009	Autonomic dysreflexia
00010	Risk for autonomic dysreflexia
00116	Disorganized infant behavior
00115	Risk for disorganized infant behavior
00117	Readiness for enhanced organized infant behavior
00049	Decreased intracranial adaptive capacity

Domain 10 Life Principles

Principles underlying conduct, thought, and behavior about acts, customs, or institutions viewed as being true or having intrinsic worth

Class 1 Values The identification and ranking of preferred modes of conduct or end states

Class 2 Beliefs Opinions, expectations, or judgments about acts, customs, or institutions viewed as being true or having intrinsic worth

Approved Diagnoses

| 00068 | Readiness for enhanced spiritual well-being |

Class 3 Value/Belief/Action Congruence The correspondence or balance achieved between values, beliefs, and actions

Approved Diagnoses

00066	Spiritual distress
00067	Risk for spiritual distress
00083	Decisional conflict (specify)

continued

Table 2.1 *continued*

00079	*Noncompliance (specify)*
00170	*Risk for impaired religiosity*
00169	*Impaired religiosity*
00171	*Readiness for enhanced religiosity*

Domain 11 Safety/Protection

Freedom from danger, physical injury, or immune system damage; preservation from loss; and protection of safety and security

Class 1 Infection Host responses following pathogenic invasion

Approved Diagnoses
00004   *Risk for infection*

Class 2 Physical Injury Bodily harm or hurt

Approved Diagnoses
00045	*Impaired oral mucous membrane*
00035	*Risk for injury*
00087	*Risk for perioperative positioning injury*
00155	*Risk for falls*
00038	*Risk for trauma*
00046	*Impaired skin integrity*
00047	*Risk for impaired skin integrity*
00044	*Impaired tissue integrity*
00048	*Impaired dentition*
00036	*Risk for suffocation*
00039	*Risk for aspiration*
00031	*Ineffective airway clearance*
00086	*Risk for peripheral neurovascular dysfunction*
00043	*Ineffective protection*
00156	*Risk for sudden infant death syndrome*

Class 3 Violence The exertion of excessive force or power so as to cause injury or abuse

Approved Diagnoses
00139	*Risk for self-mutilation*
00151	*Self-mutilation*
00138	*Risk for other-directed violence*
00140	*Risk for self-directed violence*
00150	*Risk for suicide*

Class 4 Environmental Hazards Sources of danger in the surroundings

Approved Diagnoses
00037   *Risk for poisoning*

Class 5 Defensive Processes The processes by which the self protects itself from the nonself

Approved Diagnoses
00041   *Latex allergy response*
00042   *Risk for latex allergy response*

Class 6 Thermoregulation The physiologic process of regulating heat and energy within the body for purposes of protecting the organism

Approved Diagnoses
00005   *Risk for imbalanced body temperature*
00008   *Ineffective thermoregulation*
00006   *Hypothermia*
00007   *Hyperthermia*

Domain 12 Comfort
Sense of mental, physical, or social well-being or ease

Class 1 Physical Comfort Sense of well-being or ease and/or freedom from pain

Approved Diagnoses
00132   *Acute pain*
00133   *Chronic pain*
00134   *Nausea*

Class 2 Environmental Comfort Sense of well-being or ease in/with one's environment

Class 3 Social Comfort Sense of well-being or ease with one's social situations

Approved Diagnoses
00053   *Social isolation*

Domain 13 Growth/Development
Age-appropriate increases in physical dimensions, maturation of organ systems, and/or progression through the developmental milestones

continued

Table 2.1 *continued*

Class 1 Growth Increases in physical dimensions or maturity of organ systems

Approved Diagnoses

00111	*Delayed growth and development*
00113	*Risk for disproportionate growth*
00101	*Adult failure to thrive*

Class 2 Development Progression or regression through a sequence of recognized milestones in life

Approved Diagnoses

00111	*Delayed growth and development*
00112	*Risk for delayed development*

structure was explored. The purposes of a common structure are to make visible a relationship among the three classifications—nursing diagnoses, nursing interventions, nursing outcomes—and facilitate the linkage among the three systems. The possibilities were discussed among members of the NANDA Board of Directors and the leadership of the Classification Center.

Dorothy Jones, representing NANDA, and Joanne Mc-Closkey Dochterman, representing the Classification Center, developed a funding proposal to convene an invitational conference. The proposal was funded by the National Library of Medicine, and a three-day meeting was held August 12–14, 2001, at the Starved Rock Conference Center in Utica, Illinois.

The conference brought together 24 experts in standardized nursing language development, testing, and refinement. The goal was to develop one common structure for nursing practice, including NANDA (nursing diagnoses), NIC (Nursing Intervention Classification), and NOC (Nursing Outcomes Classification), with possibilities for the inclusion of other languages as well. A detailed account of the conference, as well as the history and development, can be found in *Unifying Nursing Languages: The Harmonization of NANDA, NIC, and NOC* (Dochterman & Jones, 2003).

The NANDA Taxonomy Committee met in January 2003 to place the nursing diagnoses from *NANDA Nursing Diagnoses: Definitions and Classification, 2003–2004* into the NNN Taxonomy of Nursing Practice. The Committee established rules governing the placement of the nursing diagnoses:

1. The nursing diagnosis *definition and defining characteristics guided* the placement of the nursing diagnosis in the taxonomic structure.
2. When a nursing diagnosis *bridges two or more domains,* the Taxonomy Committee reviewed the definition and defining characteristics of the diagnosis and placed it in the domain clinically consistent with that information.
3. On review of the definition and defining characteristics of a nursing diagnosis, and if it was *clinically consistent with two or more domains,* the diagnosis was placed where the practicing nurse would expect to find that diagnosis.
4. Some nursing diagnoses *could not be placed* because there was no consensus among the members of the Taxonomy Committee. For example, *deficient diversional activity* and *delayed surgical recovery* could be placed in several domains and classes, but were left out.
5. When there is a *"risk for"* or *"readiness for enhanced"* nursing diagnosis, the Taxonomy Committee placed it in the same domain and class as the actual nursing diagnosis, when one existed.

As new nursing diagnoses are approved by NANDA International, the Taxonomy Committee will continue to place them in the NNN Taxonomy of Nursing Practice.

(text continues on page 264)

Table 2.2 NNN Taxonomy of Nursing Practice: Placement of Nursing Diagnoses

Domains	Classes	Diagnoses, Outcomes, and Interventions	NANDA Nursing Diagnoses
I. Functional Includes diagnoses, outcomes, and interventions to promote basic needs	**Activity/Exercise**	Physical activity, including energy conservation and expenditure	Activity intolerance Risk for activity intolerance Risk for disuse syndrome Risk for falls Fatigue Impaired bed mobility Impaired physical mobility Impaired wheelchair mobility Impaired transfer ability Impaired walking Sedentary lifestyle
	Comfort	A sense of emotional, physical, and spiritual well being and relative freedom from distress	Nausea Acute pain Chronic pain Energy field disturbance
	Growth and Development	Physical, emotional, and social growth and development milestones	Risk for delayed development Adult failure to thrive

		Delayed growth and development
		Risk for disproportionate growth
		Disorganized infant behavior
		Risk for disorganized infant behavior
		Readiness for enhanced organized infant behavior
Nutrition	Processes related to taking in, assimilating, and using nutrients	*Effective breastfeeding*
		Ineffective breastfeeding
		Interrupted breastfeeding
		Ineffective infant feeding pattern
		Imbalanced nutrition: Less than body requirements
		Imbalanced nutrition: More than body requirements
		Risk for imbalanced nutrition: More than body requirements
		Readiness for enhanced nutrition
		Impaired swallowing
Self-Care	Ability to accomplish basic and instrumental activities of daily living	*Bathing/hygiene self-care deficit*
		Dressing/grooming self-care deficit

continued

Table 2.2 *continued*

Domains	Classes	Diagnoses, Outcomes, and Interventions	NANDA Nursing Diagnoses
I. Functional *(continued)*			
	Sexuality	Maintenance or modification of sexual identity and patterns	*Sexual dysfunction* *Ineffective sexuality patterns*
	Sleep/Rest	The quantity and quality of sleep, rest and relaxation patterns	*Sleep deprivation* *Disturbed sleep pattern* *Readiness for enhanced sleep*
	Values/Beliefs	Ideas, goals, perceptions, spiritual and other beliefs that influence choices or decisions	*Spiritual distress* *Risk for spiritual distress* *Readiness for enhanced spiritual well-being* *Impaired religiosity* *Risk for impaired religiosity* *Readiness for enhanced religiosity*

II. Physiological Includes diagnoses, outcomes, and interventions to promote optimal biophysical health		
	Cardiac Function	Cardiac mechanisms used to maintain tissue profusion	Decreased cardiac output Ineffective tissue perfusion
	Elimination	Processes related to secretion and excretion of body wastes	Bowel incontinence Constipation Perceived constipation Risk for constipation Diarrhea Functional urinary incontinence Reflex urinary incontinence Stress urinary incontinence Total urinary incontinence Urge urinary incontinence Risk for urge urinary incontinence Impaired urinary elimination Urinary retention Readiness for enhanced urinary elimination
	Fluid & Electrolyte	Regulation of fluid/electrolytes and acid base balance	Deficient fluid volume Excess fluid volume Risk for deficient fluid volume Risk for imbalanced fluid volume Readiness for enhanced fluid balance

continued

Table 2.2 *continued*

Domains	*Classes*	*Diagnoses, Outcomes, and Interventions*	*NANDA Nursing Diagnoses*
II. Physiological *(continued)*	**Neurocognition**	Mechanisms related to the nervous system and neurocognitive functioning, including memory, thinking, and judgment	Autonomic dysreflexia Risk for autonomic dysreflexia Acute confusion Chronic confusion Impaired environmental interpretation syndrome Decreased intracranial adaptive capacity Impaired memory Unilateral neglect Disturbed thought processes Wandering
	Pharmacological Function	Effects (therapeutic and adverse) of medications or drugs and other pharmacologically active products	

Physical Regulation Body temperature, endocrine, and immune system responses to regulate cellular processes

Latex allergy response
Risk for latex allergy response
Risk for imbalanced body temperature
Hyperthermia
Hypothermia
Risk for infection
Risk for peripheral neurovascular dysfunction
Ineffective protection
ineffective thermoregulation

Reproduction Processes related to human procreation and birth

Ineffective airway clearance
Risk for aspiration
Ineffective breathing pattern
Impaired gas exchange
Risk for suffocation
Impaired spontaneous ventilation
Dysfunctional ventilatory weaning response

Respiratory Function Ventilation adequate to maintain arterial blood gases within normal limits

Disturbed sensory perception

continued

Table 2.2 continued

Domains	Classes	Diagnoses, Outcomes, and Interventions	NANDA Nursing Diagnoses
II. Physiological (continued)	**Sensation/Perception**	Intake and interpretation of information through the senses, including seeing, hearing, touching, tasting, smelling	Impaired dentition Impaired oral mucous membrane Impaired skin integrity Risk for impaired skin integrity Impaired tissue integrity
	Tissue Integrity	Skin and mucous membrane protection to support secretion, excretion, and healing	Ineffective health maintenance Health-seeking behaviors Noncompliance
III. Psychosocial Includes diagnoses, outcomes, and interventions to promote optimal mental and emotional health and social functioning	**Behavior**	Actions that promote, maintain, or restore health	Ineffective therapeutic regimen management Ineffective community therapeutic regimen management Ineffective family therapeutic regimen management Readiness for enhanced therapeutic regimen management

Communication	Receiving, interpreting, and expressing spoken, written, and nonverbal messages	*Impaired verbal communication* *Readiness for enhanced communication*
Coping	Adjusting or adapting to stressful events	*Impaired adjustment* *Decisional conflict* *Ineffective coping* *Ineffective community coping* *Readiness for enhanced community coping* *Defensive coping* *compromised family coping* *Disabled family coping* *Readiness for enhanced family coping* *Ineffective denial* *Anticipatory grieving* *Dysfunctional grieving* *Risk for dysfunctional grieving* *Post-trauma syndrome* *Risk for post-trauma syndrome* *Rape-trauma syndrome* *Rape-trauma syndrome: Compound reaction*

continued

Table 2.2 *continued*

Domains	Classes	Diagnoses, Outcomes, and Interventions	NANDA Nursing Diagnoses
III. Psychosocial *(continued)*			*Rape-trauma syndrome: Silent reaction*
			Relocation stress syndrome
			Risk for relocation stress syndrome
			Self-mutilation
			Risk for self-mutilation
			Risk for suicide
			Risk for self-directed violence
			Readiness for enhanced coping
	Emotional	A mental state or feeling that may influence perceptions of the world	*Anxiety*
			Death anxiety
			Fear
			Hopelessness
			Chronic sorrow
	Knowledge	Understanding and skill in applying information to promote, maintain, and restore health	*Deficient knowledge (specify)*
			Readiness for enhanced knowledge (specify)

Roles/Relationships	Maintenance and/or modification of expected social behaviors and emotional connectedness with others	*Risk for impaired parent/infant/ child attachment* *Caregiver role strain* *Risk for caregiver role strain* *Parental role conflict* *Dysfunctional family processes: Alcoholism* *Interrupted family processes* *Impaired parenting* *Risk for impaired parenting* *Ineffective role performance* *Impaired social interaction* *Social isolation* *Risk for other-directed violence* *Readiness for enhanced family processes* *Readiness for enhanced parenting*
Self-Perception	Awareness of one's body and personal identity	*Disturbed body image* *Disturbed personal identity* *Risk for loneliness* *Powerlessness*

continued

Table 2.2 *continued*

Domains	Classes	Diagnoses, Outcomes, and Interventions	NANDA Nursing Diagnoses
III. Psychosocial *(continued)*			*Risk for powerlessness* *Chronic low self-esteem* *Situational low self-esteem* *Risk for situational low self-esteem* *Readiness for enhanced self-concept*
IV. Environmental Includes diagnoses, outcomes, and interventions to promote and protect the environmental health and safety of individuals, systems, and communities	**Healthcare System**	Social, political, and economic structures and processes for the delivery of health-care services	
	Populations	Aggregates of individuals or communities having characteristics in common	
	Risk Management	Avoidance of identifiable health threats	*Impaired home maintenance* *Risk for injury* *Risk for perioperative positioning injury* *Risk for poisoning*

Risk for trauma
Risk for sudden infant death syndrome

Unable to place in the structure:
Deficient diversional activity
Delayed surgical recovery

Further Development of Taxonomy II

A multiaxial framework allows clinicians to see where there are gaps and/or potentially useful new diagnoses. If you construct a new diagnosis or a set of diagnoses that is useful to your practice, please submit it (them) to NANDA so others can share in the discovery. Submission guidelines are on page 269; submission forms can be found on the NANDA Web site (www.nanda.org). Concept analysis methods and NANDA submission forms can be found on the NLINKS Web site (www.nlinks.org). The Diagnostic Review Committee will be glad to help you prepare the submission. For assistance and/or questions, contact committee chair Leann Scroggins (scroggins.leann@mayo.edu) or the NANDA office at 1211 Locust Street, Philadelphia, PA 19107. Telephone: 800.647.9002 or 215.545.8105; fax, 215.545.8107.

References

Braham, C. G., & the Random House Reference Staff (Eds.). (1998). *Random House Webster's dictionary* (3rd ed.). New York: Ballantine Books.

Coenen, A., McNeil, B., Bakken, S., Bickford, C., & Warren, J. (2001). Toward comparable nursing data: American Nurses Association criteria for data sets, classification systems, and nomenclatures. *Computers in Nursing, 19,* 240–248.

Dochterman, J., & Jones, D. (Eds.). (2003). *Unifying nursing languages: The harmonization of NANDA, NIC, and NOC.* Washington, DC: American Nurses Association.

Gordon. M. (1998). *Manual of nursing diagnosis.* St. Louis: Mosby.

Jenny, J. (1994). Advancing the science of nursing with nursing diagnosis. In M. Rantz & P. LeMone (Eds.), *Classification of nursing diagnoses: Proceedings of the eleventh conference* (pp. 73–81). Glendale, CA: CINAHL.

Johnson, M.., & Maas, M. (1997). *Nursing outcomes classification (NOC).* St. Louis: Mosby.

NANDA. (1991). The NANDA definition of nursing diagnosis. In R.M. Carroll-Johnson (Ed.), Classifications of nursing diagnosis: Proceedings of the ninth conference (pp. 65–71). Philadelphia: Lippincott.

NANDA. (1999). *NANDA nursing diagnoses: Definitions & classification 1999–2000.* Philadelphia: Author.

NANDA. (2000). *NANDA nursing diagnoses: Definitions & classification 2001–2002.* Philadelphia: Author.

Roget's II: The New Thesaurus. (1980). Boston: Houghton Mifflin.

Part 3

NURSING DIAGNOSIS DEVELOPMENT

2005–2006

Diagnosis Submission Guidelines
Protocol for Submission or Revision of Diagnoses

Proposed diagnoses and revisions of diagnoses undergo a systematic review to determine consistency with the established criteria for a nursing diagnosis. All submissions are subsequently staged according to evidence supporting either the level of development or validation.

Diagnoses may be submitted at various levels of development (e.g., label and definition; label, definition, defining characteristics or risk factors, related factors). Any submission beyond that of label and definition must include an integrative review of the relevant nursing literature. If no nursing literature is available, please indicate this in the literature review. Related research from other disciplines is also appropriate to include. *NANDA Guidelines for Nursing Diagnosis Submission* and forms are available from the NANDA office, on the NANDA International Web site (www.nanda.org), and the NLINKS Web site (www.nlinks.org; click on "diagnostic review"). Articles used for the submission are to be catalogued on a Literature Review Form (see submission/review packet).

E-mail your submission to nanda@rmpinc.org or mail a CD to NANDA International at 1211 Locust Street, Philadelphia, PA 19107, USA. All diagnoses are to be submitted in the format provided in the packet. The submitter is asked to compare his/her submission with all current related NANDA diagnoses (see example in submission/review packet).

On receipt, the diagnosis will be assigned to a primary reviewer from the Diagnosis Review Committee (DRC). This person will work with you as the DRC reviews your submission. Once the diagnosis is formally reviewed by the DRC, it will be sent to nursing specialty group experts and the NANDA International Committee for comment. Recommendations will be shared with you. Diagnoses will then be discussed in forums at the next NANDA biennial conference in order to invite extended member input. Recommendations from the forums will be reviewed and the diagnoses forwarded to the NANDA International Board of Directors. All diagnoses accepted at the 2.1 level of development will be included in the next edition of *NANDA Nursing Diagnoses: Definitions & Classification*.

NANDA Diagnosis Submission: PRELIMINARY STEPS

To submit a diagnosis for consideration by the DRC:

1. Obtain the most recent edition of *NANDA Nursing Diagnoses: Definitions and Classification* and review the "NANDA Diagnosis Submission Guidelines." These guidelines are also accessible on the NANDA Web site (www.nanda.org; click on "NANDA Diagnosis Submission") and on the NLINKS Web site (www.nlinks.org; click on "diagnostic review").

2. Contact Leann Scroggins (scroggins.leann@mayo.edu), Chair of the Diagnosis Review Committee, for more specific instructions, guidelines regarding format, criteria for assigning level of evidence, and protocol for submission.

3. Review "Glossary of Terms" in the same edition of *NANDA Nursing Diagnoses: Definitions and Classification*.

4. Decide whether your diagnosis is an actual diagnosis, a risk diagnosis, or a wellness diagnosis.

5. Provide a label for the diagnosis.

6. Provide a definition for the diagnosis that is supported by references.

7. Identify the defining characteristics or risk factors for the diagnosis. References (articles, not books) to back up each defining characteristic or risk factor are required.

The references should be research-based if possible. If no research-based references or nursing references are available, indicate this in your submission.

8. Identify related factors and provide references for each one.

9. Develop a bibliography, including all the articles you referenced. In addition, identify the three key references you want to be included in *NANDA Nursing Diagnoses: Definitions & Classification* when your submission is accepted.

10. E-mail the above to nanda@rmpinc.org, and mail a paper copy of all the referenced articles to NANDA International, 1211 Locust Street, Philadelphia, PA, 19107, USA.

11. You will be notified when your work has been received and will be given an estimate of the time it will take before you can expect to receive a response from the DRC. Most submissions need some additional work or refinement. You will be assigned a mentor from the Diagnosis Review Committee to assist you through the process.

NANDA Diagnosis Submission: Level of Evidence Criteria

1 Received for Development (Consultation from DRC)

1.1 Label Only
This level is primarily intended for submission by organized groups rather than individuals. The DRC will consult with and educate potential developers through distribution of printed guidelines for diagnostic development experts. At this stage the label would be categorized as "received for development."

1.2 Label and Definition

The label is clear and stated at a basic level. The definition is consistent with the label. The label and definition should be distinct and contrast from other diagnoses. The definition differs from the defining characteristics and label, and these components should not be included in the definition. At this stage, the diagnosis must be consistent with the current NANDA definition of nursing diagnosis; it will be screened for meeting this criterion.

1.3 Label, Definition, and Defining Characteristics or Risk Factors

The defining characteristics or risk factors (for risk diagnoses) should be consistent with the label. The defining characteristics should be distinct, observable, and measurable. The list of defining characteristics may include both major and minor characteristics. The number of major characteristics should be limited to 5-7.

1.4 Label, Definition, Defining Characteristics or Risk Factors, References

The label, definition, and defining characteristics are consistent. References are included. Criteria 1.2 and 1.3 must be met. At stages 1.2, 1.3, and 1.4, the content will be examined for consistency with the current nursing knowledge base. The content should be consistent with all NANDA definitions and qualifiers. Collaboration with experts may be utilized. Consultation with DRC is encouraged.

2 Accepted for Publication and Inclusion in the NANDA Taxonomy

2.1 Label, Definition, Defining Characteristics or Risk Factors, Related Factors, References, and Literature Review

At 2.1, the label will be forwarded to the Taxonomy Committee for classification. A narrative review of relevant literature, culminating in a written concept analysis, is required to demonstrate the existence of a substantive body of knowledge underlying the diagnosis. The literature review/concept analysis should support the label and definition. It should also include discussion and support of the defining characteristics or risk factors (for risk diagnoses) and related factors (for actual diagnoses).

2.2 Consensus Studies Related to Diagnosis Using Nurse Experts

The criteria in 2.1 are met. Studies include opinionnaire, Delphi, and similar studies of diagnostic components in which nurses are subjects.

3 Clinically Supported (Validation and Testing)

3.1 Literature Synthesis

The criteria in 2.1 are met. The synthesis is in the form of an integrated review of the literature. Search terms/MESH terms used in the review are provided to assist future researchers.

3.2 Clinical Studies Related to Diagnosis, But Not Generalizable to the Population

The criteria in 2.1 are met. The narrative includes a description of studies related to the diagnosis, which includes defining characteristics or risk factors, and related factors. Studies may be qualitative in nature, or quantitative studies using nonrandom samples in which patients are subjects.

3.3   Well-Designed Clinical Studies With Small Sample Sizes

The criteria in 2.1 are met. The narrative includes a description of studies related to the diagnosis, which includes defining characteristics or risk factors. Random sampling is used in these studies, but sample size is limited.

3.4   Well-Designed Clinical Studies With Random Sample of Sufficient Size to Allow for Generalizability to the Overall Population

The criteria in 2.1 are met. The narrative includes a description of studies related to the diagnosis, which includes defining characteristics or risk factors, and related factors. Random sampling is used in these studies, sample size is sufficient to allow for generalizability of results to the overall population.

Procedure to Appeal a DRC Decision on Diagnosis Review

If a diagnosis/revision is reviewed by the DRC and returned to the submitter(s) either for revision or because it is judged not to meet one or more criteria for staging a diagnosis, the submitter(s) may appeal the decision.

If the DRC chooses not to accept a diagnosis/revision, notification of nonacceptance will be given to the submitter(s) with detailed rationale. One or more of the following reasons will be explained:

- Reject diagnosis (e.g., does not meet criteria for the definition of a nursing diagnosis or does not meet diagnosis level of evidence criteria)
- Return with substantial revision (e.g., need to make major content changes)
- Insufficient/old literature support (e.g., failure to reference meta analyses, concept papers, current research, or lack of research articles)
- Return with editorial changes (e.g., solicit submitter response to DRC rationale and/or revision to submission)

If the submitter(s) choose(s) to appeal the DRC decision, the proposed diagnosis/revision will be placed on the NANDA International Web site (www.nanda.org) and will be announced in the journal. A period of 90 days will be provided for members to submit evidence supporting, modifying, or rejecting the diagnosis/revision. After 90 days, the DRC will review feedback and submit a second decision to the submitter(s).

If the DRC once again chooses not to accept a diagnosis/revision, the submitter(s) will have an opportunity at the biennial conference to present the diagnosis/revision and the rationale for disagreement with the DRC decision. The presentation to DRC would occur in open session and require evidence-based argument regarding the DRC decision. Other members will also be able to present evidence supporting, modifying, or rejecting the diagnosis/revision. At the end of this time, the DRC will review all information and submit a decision to the submitter and the Board of Directors prior to the end of the conference.

The NANDA International Board of Directors will have an opportunity to provide evidence-based argument supporting, modifying, or rejecting the submission at four points:

1. After the initial DRC review
2. After the final review of the 2-year cycle and prior to the conference
3. If there is an appeal, the Board will have the opportunity to provide the DRC with evidence to support, reject, or modify the diagnosis/revision before DRC makes its final recommendation prior to the end of the conference
4. After the conference, the NANDA International Board of Directors votes on all diagnoses/ revisions, which provides a final review. If the board continues to have reservations about a diagnosis/revision, it may request the DRC to solicit further information from the submitter(s) prior to approval of the diagnosis. This ensures that each diagnosis is held to the same standard for review and that decisions are made on the basis of evidence/research rather than opinion.

Glossary of Terms

Nursing Diagnoses

Nursing diagnosis A clinical judgment about individual, family, or community responses to actual or potential health problems/life processes. A nursing diagnosis provides the basis for selection of nursing interventions to achieve outcomes for which the nurse is accountable (approved at the 9th conference, 1990).

Actual nursing diagnosis Describes human responses to health conditions/life processes that exist in an individual, family, or community. It is supported by defining characteristics (manifestations, signs and symptoms) that cluster in patterns of related cues or inferences.

Risk nursing diagnosis Describes human responses to health conditions/life processes that may develop in a vulnerable individual, family, or community. It is supported by risk factors that contribute to increased vulnerability.

Syndrome "A cluster or group of signs and symptoms that almost always occur together. Together, these clusters represent a distinct clinical picture" (McCourt, 1991, p. 79).

Wellness nursing diagnosis Describes human responses to levels of wellness in an individual, family, or community that have a readiness for enhancement.

Components of a Diagnosis

Label Provides a name for a diagnosis. It is a concise term or phrase that represents a pattern of related cues. It may include modifiers.

Definition Provides a clear, precise description; delineates its meaning and helps differentiate it from similar diagnoses.

Defining characteristics Observable cues/inferences that cluster as manifestations of an actual or wellness nursing diagnosis.

Risk factors Environmental factors and physiological, psychological, genetic, or chemical elements that increase the vulnerability of an individual, family, or community to an unhealthful event.

Related factors Factors that appear to show some type of patterned relationship with the nursing diagnosis. Such factors may be described as antecedent to, associated with, related to, contributing to, or abetting.

Definitions for Classification of Nursing Diagnoses

Classification Systematic arrangement of related phenomena in groups or classes based on characteristics that objects have in common

Level of abstraction Describes the concreteness/abstractness of a concept:

(a) Very abstract concepts are theoretical, may not be directly measurable, defined by concrete concepts, inclusive of concrete concepts, disassociated from any specific instance, independent of time and space, have more general descriptors, may not be clinically useful for planning treatment.

(b) Concrete concepts are observable and measurable, limited by time and space, constitute a specific category, more exclusive, name a real thing or class of things, restricted by nature, may be clinically useful for planning treatment.

Nomenclature A system of designations (terms) elaborated according to pre-established rules (American Nurses Association, 1999)

Taxonomy Classification according to presumed natural relationships among types and their subtypes (American Nurses Association, 1999).

Reference

American Nurses Association. (1999). *ANA CNP II recognition criteria and definitions.* Washington, DC: Author.

McCourt, A. (1991). In R.M. Carroll-Johnson (Ed.), *Classification of nursing diagnoses: Proceedings of the ninth conference* (p. 79). Philadelphia: Lippincott.

NANDA Guidelines for Copyright Permission

The materials presented in this book are copyrighted and all copyright laws apply. Situations requiring approvals and/or copyright fees are listed below:

1. An author or publishing house requests use of the entire nursing diagnosis taxonomy in a textbook or other nursing manual to be sold.
2. An author or publishing house requests use of only the list of nursing diagnoses with no definitions or defining characteristics.
3. An author or company requests use of the nursing diagnosis taxonomy in an audiovisual material.
4. A software developer or computer-based patient record vendor requests use of the nursing diagnosis taxonomy in a program.
5. A nursing school, researcher, professional organization, or healthcare organization requests use of the nursing diagnosis taxonomy in a program.

Send all permission requests to
NANDA International
1211 Locust St.
Philadelphia, PA 19107, USA
phone: 800.647.9002/215.545.7222
fax: 215.545.8107
e-mail: nanda@rmpinc.com.

2004–2006

NANDA International Board of Directors

President: Martha Craft Rosenberg, PhD, RN, FAAN
President-Elect: T. Heather Herdman, PhD, RN
Secretary: Rona F. Levin, PhD, RN
Treasurer: Anne Perry, EdD, RN, FAAN
Directors:
   Dame June Clark, PhD, RN, RHV, FRNC, DBE
   Barbara Krainovich-Miller, EdD, RN
   Dickon Weir-Hughes, EdD, RN, FRSH

NANDA International Diagnosis Review Committee

Leann Scroggins, MSN, RN, *Chair*
Davina Gosnell, PhD, RN, FAAN
Marlene Lindeman, MSN, RN, CS
Lynda Juall Carpenito-Moyet, MSN, RN, CRNP
Geralyn Meyer, PhD, RN
Jean O'Neil, EdD, RN
Linal Rahal, RN
Dorothy Jones, EdD, RN, FAAN
Meridean Maas, PhD, RN, FAAN
T. Heather Herdman, PhD, RN, *Board Liaison*
Barbara Krainovich-Miller, EdD, RN, *Board Liaison*

NANDA International Taxonomy Committee

Barbara Vassallo, EdD, RN, CS, ANPC, *Chair*
Marion Johnson, PhD, RN
Judy Myers, MSN, RN
Christy Paul, MEd, RNC
Dame June Clark, PhD, RN, RHV, FRNC, DBE

Nursing Diagnosis Extension and Classification (NDEC) Research Team

Principal Investigator
Martha Craft-Rosenberg, PhD, RN, FAAN

NDEC Investigators
Noriko Abe, MA, RN
Judy Collins, MA, RN
Hyun-Wook Kang, MA, RN
Aaran Lee, MA, RN
Megan McGonigal-Kenny, MA, RN

2002–2004

NANDA Board of Directors

President: Mary Ann Lavin, ScD, RN, CS, ANP, FAAN
President-Elect: Martha Craft-Rosenberg, PhD, RN, FAAN
Secretary: Rona Levin, PhD, RN
Treasurer: Sheila Sparks Ralph, DNSc, RN, FAAN
Directors:
   Kay Avant, PhD, RN, FAAN
   T. Heather Herdman, PhD, RN
   Anne Perry, EdD, RN
   Dickon Weir-Hughes, EdD, RN, FRSH
   Georgia Griffith Whitley, EdD, RN

NANDA Diagnosis Review Committee

Leann Scroggins, MSN, RN, *Co-Chair*
Davina Gosnell, PhD, RN, FAAN, *Co-Chair*
Marlene Lindeman, MSN, RN, CS
Lynda Juall Carpenito-Moyet, MSN, RN, CRNP
Geralyn Meyer, PhD, RN
Jean O'Neil, EdD, RN
Lina Rahal, RN
T. Heather Herdman, PhD, RN, *Board Liaison*

NANDA Taxonomy Committee

Barbara Vassallo, EdD, RN, CS, ANPC, *Co-Chair*
Rose Harvey, DNSc, RN, *Co-Chair*
June Clark, PhD, RN, FHU, FRCN
Judy Myers, MSN, RN
Marion Johnson, PhD, RN
Martha Craft-Rosenberg, PhD, RN, FAAN, *Board Liaison*

Nursing Diagnosis Extension and Classification (NDEC) Research Team

Principal Investigator
Martha Craft-Rosenberg, PhD, RN, FAAN

NDEC Investigators
Lisa Burkhart, PhD, RN
Dame June Clark, DBE, PhD, RN, RHV, FRNC
Mary Clarke, MA, RN
Judith A. Collins, MA, ARNP, CNS
Connie Delaney, PhD, RN, FAAN
Gloria Dorr, MA, ARNP
Theresa Gibbs, MA, ARNP
Cyd Q. Grafft, MS, RN, ARNP
Kathleen Hanson, PhD, RN
Scott Lamount, MS, RN, ARNP
Aeran Lee, MS, RN
Lucina Sheehy, MS., RN
Janet Specht, PhD, RN, FAAN
Jane Tang, MS, RN

Chair, NDEC Satellite Groups
Mary Jane Oakland, PhD, RD, LD, FADA

An Invitation to Join NANDA International

Mission

To advance the development of nursing terminologies and classifications and provide nurses at all levels of practice with a standardized language to:

- Assess client responses to actual or potential health problems or life crises,
- Document care for reimbursement of nursing services by third party insurers, and
- Create and use databases that facilitate documentation and the study of the phenomena of concern to nurses in order to improve patient care.

Functions

1. Provide nurses with a standardized language describing their practice that can be used to communicate with nurses across all specialties and cultures, members of other healthcare disciplines, and the healthcare consumer.
2. Provide a system for developing, validating, and refining nursing terminologies and classifications.
3. Publish a quarterly journal that contains the latest thinking about nursing terminologies and classifications worldwide.
4. Provide support, communication, and resources through conferences, publications, funding, and networking. Mentoring is available for nurses who are interested in developing new diagnoses and refining current diagnoses.

Membership Requirements

Membership is open to all registered nurses with a current RN license. Associate membership is extended to nonregistered nurses and students who share an interest in the purpose of the association. Institutional membership is extended to those associations and organizations that believe in and want to support the mission of NANDA International.

Organizational Background

The North American Nursing Diagnosis Association (NANDA) was founded in 1982, replacing the National Conference Group that was established in 1973. In 2002 the association name was changed to NANDA International to reflect its worldwide expansion. To date, NANDA has approved 172 diagnoses for clinical testing and refinement.

A dynamic process of diagnosis review and taxonomy development continues toward identifying and classifying nursing phenomena. NANDA-approved diagnoses are included in the Unified Medical Language System of the National Library of Medicine and Health Level 7 (HL7), and NANDA is working with the American Nurses Association to develop a Unified Nursing Language System. NANDA is also cooperating with the International Council of Nurses to develop an International Classification of Nursing Practice.

Benefits of Membership

1. Subscription to the *International Journal of Nursing Terminologies and Classifications*
2. Reduced registration fee at the NNN biennial conference.
3. Participation in decisions about new and revised diagnoses.
4. State-of-the-art information on development of nursing language systems, which enable nurses to communicate with one another around the world.
5. Reduced rate on in-house publications, such as *Nursing Diagnoses: Definitions & Classification.*
6. Resources for networking and research data.
7. Access to the NANDA Web page with links to minutes from the Board of Director meetings and all current decisions and initiatives.

Additional Materials Available

NANDA publishes its taxonomy in *NANDA Nursing Diagnoses: Definitions and Classification.* A new edition is printed after each biennial conference. This book contains the only list of diagnoses approved by NANDA for distribution.

To order or obtain information on NANDA publications or conferences, contact the NANDA office:
1211 Locust St., Philadelphia, PA 19107.
800.647.9002; E-mail: NANDA@nursecominc.com;
Web: www.nanda.org

Membership Committee

Scott Lamont, RN, CCRN, CFRN, ENCC, *Co-Chair*
Mary Ann Lavin, ScD, RN, BC, ANP, FAAN, *Co-Chair*
Eleanor Borkowski, BSN, RN
Lisa Burkhart, PhD, RN
Marjory Gordon, PhD, RN, FAAN
Margaret McComb, MSN, RN
Mercedes Ugalde Apalategui, MHS, RN
Dickon Weir-Hughes, EdD, RN, FRSH, *Board Liaison*

☐ YES! I WANT TO SUPPORT THE NURSING TERMINOLOGY MOVEMENT. PLEASE ACCEPT MY APPLICATION FOR NANDA INTERNATIONAL MEMBERSHIP:

☐ Regular Membership (RNs only)...US $100*
☐ Retired Membership ....US $ 65*
☐ Associate Membership (non-RNs welcome) ....US $100*
☐ Student Membership ....US $ 29*
(Open to matriculating undergraduate students. Proof of enrollment required; limited to 3 years.)

Institutional membership is also available. Contact our office for details.
☐ Send ___copy(ies) of *NANDA Nursing Diagnoses*: $_____
Definitions & Classification at special member's price:
US $15.95/ea.
☐ Send ___copy(ies) of *Critical Thinking & Nursing* $_____
Diagnoses at special member's price: US $19.95/ea.
☐ I am also enclosing my tax-deductible donation to $_____
the NANDA Foundation

TOTAL ENCLOSED ....US $_____

NANDA's Federal Tax ID # is 41-1363777.

☐ Check enclosed   ☐ Money order enclosed
(Payable to NANDA. US funds drawn on US banks only)
☐ Charge my credit card: ☐ AmEx   ☐ MC   ☐ Visa
CARD # _____
Signature_____ Exp. date___/___

* US $29 of this amount is for your one-year subscription to the *International Journal of Nursing Terminologies & Classifications*.

PLEASE PRINT

_____
FIRST NAME   M.I.

_____
LAST NAME & CREDENTIALS

_____
CURRENT LICENSE NUMBER

_____
POSITION/TITLE(S)

_____
COMPANY/INSTITUTION

_____
DEPARTMENT

_____
MAILING ADDRESS (PREFERRED) _ HOME   _ BUSINESS

_____
CITY

_____
STATE/PROVINCE   ZIP/POSTAL CODE   COUNTRY

_____
TELEPHONE   FAX

_____
E-MAIL ADDRESS

Index

Notes

Notes